Point of Care Ultrasound Made Easy

T0186350

Point of Care Ultrasound Made Easy

Edited by
John McCafferty
James M Forsyth

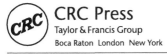

CRC Press
Taylor & Francis Group
Boca Raton London New York

CRC Press is an imprint of the
Taylor & Francis Group, an **informa** business

CRC Press
Taylor & Francis Group
6000 Broken Sound Parkway NW, Suite 300
Boca Raton, FL 33487-2742

© 2020 by Taylor & Francis Group, LLC
CRC Press is an imprint of Taylor & Francis Group, an Informa business

No claim to original U.S. Government works

Printed on acid-free paper

International Standard Book Number-13: 978-0-367-34958-5 (Paperback)
978-0-367-36601-8 (Hardback)

Library of Congress Control Number: 2020930237

Visit the Taylor & Francis Web site at
http://www.taylorandfrancis.com

and the CRC Press Web site at
http://www.crcpress.com

We dedicate this book to all busy clinicians across the world. You all work tirelessly, go beyond the call of duty every day and do make a positive difference. Ultrasound is a tool that we believe is at your disposal and can make your life easier, yet perhaps you feel you are not the right person to be using it. Well, we say otherwise and encourage you to embrace the point-of-care ultrasound revolution. We hope that you find this material helpful and that it will make a long-term positive impact on your clinical practice and ultimately lead to improved patient care.

CONTENTS

FOREWORD

This book is an easy-to-read introductory text describing the use of point-of-care ultrasound for an increasingly wide range of ultrasound applications. The book is aimed at clinicians and practitioners who are perhaps not as familiar with the use of ultrasound for diagnosis as clinical ultrasonographers and radiologists. Each chapter has concise learning objectives, and the text is punctuated with many clear and easy-to-follow diagrams illustrating scanning positions and the ultrasound images acquired at each of these positions. This will enable even the relatively novice practitioner to develop the skills necessary to obtain high-quality and focussed diagnostic information to answer fundamental clinical questions.

The publication of this book is timely as we enter an era where the use of hand-held and laptop-sized ultrasound scanners is becoming increasingly commonplace within our hospitals. This book, edited by Dr John McCafferty, a respiratory consultant at the Royal Infirmary of Edinburgh, Scotland, with a wealth of clinical experience, and Mr James M Forsyth, senior vascular surgery registrar and author of *Venous Access Made Easy*, provides clear guidance on the use and diagnostic importance of point-of-care ultrasound.

Professor Carmel Moran
Chair of Translational Ultrasound
University of Edinburgh

ACKNOWLEDGEMENTS

This book would not have been possible without our excellent team of authors (Nick, Shirjel, Anoop and Kirsten). You are all consummate professionals, expert clinicians, reliable and trustworthy colleagues and tremendously enthusiastic medical educators. You produced some excellent chapters in a very timely manner, and it was a joy to work with you all. A book like this cannot be authoritatively written by one clinician alone, and you should all be applauded for your tremendous contributions. Additional thanks must go to Professor John Murchison who contributed majorly in providing the ultrasound images used throughout the book and for his expert oversight.

In particular, I am indebted to my fellow editor John McCafferty for his expert input and tireless enthusiasm to help promote point-of-care ultrasound education. This book was originally your idea and therefore you should take full credit for its inception.

It is also great to be working with the fantastic Miranda Bromage and Samantha Cook from CRC Press/Taylor & Francis. You are a great publishing team, and it is an honour to be working with you again so soon after *Venous Access Made Easy*.

James M Forsyth

CONTRIBUTORS

Shirjel R Alam, MBChB, MRCP, MRCS, MRCA, PhD
Consultant Cardiologist
Manchester University NHS Foundation Trust
Wythenshawe Hospital
Manchester, United Kingdom

James M Forsyth, MBBS, MRCS, MSc (HPE)
Vascular and Endovascular Surgery Registrar
Leeds Vascular Institute
Leeds, United Kingdom

Kirsten MS Kind, MBChB (Edin), FRCR
Consultant Paediatric Radiologist
Royal Manchester Children's Hospital
Manchester, United Kingdom

John McCafferty, BEng, PhD, MBChB, MD, MRCP
Respiratory Consultant
Royal Infirmary of Edinburgh
Scotland, United Kingdom

John Murchison, MBChB, BSc, DMRD, FRCP, FRCR, PhD
Consultant Radiologist
Royal Infirmary of Edinburgh
and
President, Scottish Radiological Society
Scotland, United Kingdom

Anoop SV Shah, MbChB, PhD, MPH
Senior Lecturer in Cardiology
University of Edinburgh
Edinburgh, United Kingdom

Nick B Spath, MBBS, BSc, MRCP
Cardiology Registrar
NHS Lothian and Fife
Scotland, United Kingdom

PART I

BACKGROUND TO POINT-OF-CARE ULTRASOUND MADE EASY (POCUSME)

CHAPTER 1

HOW DOES ULTRASOUND WORK?

John McCafferty

Learning Objectives

- Understand the basic physics behind medical ultrasound imaging.
- Understand the hardware components of a medical ultrasound scanner.
- Understand the different imaging modes: B-mode, M-mode and Doppler.
- Know how to acquire an ultrasound image, appreciating the imaging conventions.
- Know how to optimise your ultrasound image.
- Appreciate your choices of point-of-care ultrasound (POCUS) device.
- Have an awareness of safety factors in POCUS.

What Is Ultrasound?

Ultrasound waves are mechanical energy that are transmitted through a medium from repetitive periodic oscillations of a transducer. The number of such cycles per second is termed the frequency of the ultrasound signal. Ultrasound refers to sound propagated at frequencies higher than the audible spectrum for humans (>20 KHz) (see **Figure 1.1**). Typically, medical ultrasound imaging operates in the range 3.5–20 MHz.

3

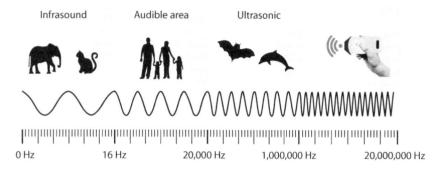

Figure 1.1 The frequency spectrum of sound waves with reference to the medical ultrasound range.

Properties of Ultrasound in Tissues

A B-mode ultrasound image is constructed from echoes generated by reflection of ultrasound from boundaries and scattering from small inhomogeneities within the tissue structures. Reflection occurs at the boundaries between two mediums of different acoustic impedance such as those between organs. Here, acoustic impedance is defined as the product of density of the tissue and the speed of sound within the tissue. The amplitude of the ultrasound wave that is reflected back into the tissue/organ or transmitted across a tissue/organ boundary is dependent on the change in acoustic impedance. If the change is small, the majority of the ultrasound will be transmitted and little reflected; if the change is large, the majority will be reflected back

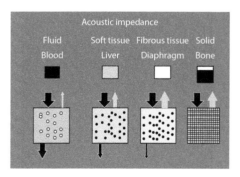

Material	Velocity of sound (m/s)	Impedance (Rayl × 10⁶)
Air	330	0.0004
Fat	1450	1.38
Water	1480	1.48
Average soft tissue	1540	1.63
Brain	1540	NA
Liver	1580	1.65
Kidney	1560	1.62
Blood	1570	1.61
Muscle	1580	1.7
Lens of eye	1620	NA
Skull bone	4080	7.8

Figure 1.2 Impedance values of typical tissues seen in the body. Air has very low impedance, meaning the ultrasound wave is strongly reflected at an air/tissue interface. This is why ultrasound gel is used when scanning a patient to avoid air interfaces between the transducer and the patient's skin.

and little transmitted. For example, the medium of fluid or water has low impedance and will conduct the ultrasound wave, whereas bone is a poor conductor and will reflect the ultrasound wave back towards its source (see **Figure 1.2**).

Small inhomogeneities within tissues/organs result in scattering of the ultrasound beam. This scattering is dependent on the size of the scatterer relative to the frequency/wavelength of the ultrasound beam. However, the scattering from these small structures (including red blood cells) is much smaller than typical reflections from boundaries so that within a B-mode image, boundaries are associated with brighter echoes compared to the less bright echoes generated by scattering within soft tissue.

Ultrasound Imaging

Ultrasound imaging uses the differences in the acoustic properties of tissues to build a picture of the structures within the body. The ultrasound signal is generated by a transducer that contains an array of tiny piezoelectric crystals which when excited by an electrical signal vibrate at a set frequency and transmit an ultrasound signal. The transducer is also a receiver, detecting the reflected signal via the piezoelectric crystals whilst 'listening' between transmission phases. This is referred to as send-receive mode (see **Figure 1.3**). The reflected signal is processed so that high intensity signals from reflected ultrasound waves represent brighter areas on screen. Complex signal processing therefore allows the display in real time of the ultrasound image as a grey-scale image on screen (see **Figure 1.4**).

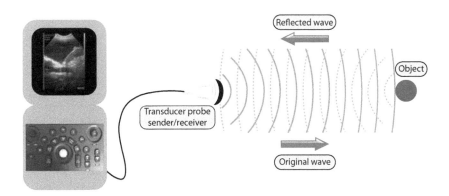

Figure 1.3 Schematic illustrating the principle of the operation of an ultrasound transducer as both an emitter and receiver of ultrasound signals.

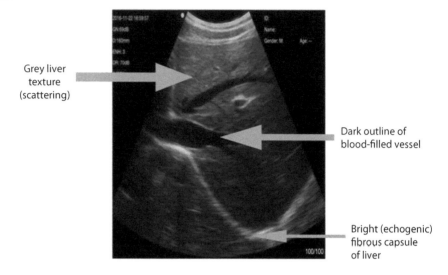

Grey liver texture (scattering)

Dark outline of blood-filled vessel

Bright (echogenic) fibrous capsule of liver

Figure 1.4 Ultrasound image of liver illustrating the grey liver texture (scattering), bright outline of the liver capsule (boundary reflection) and the dark (fluid-filled) vessel.

Image Acquisition

The ultrasound probe houses the transducer which is constructed from an array of elements and can be arranged in linear, curvilinear or phased array formats (see **Figure 1.5**). There are new technologies where the piezoelectric crystals are replaced with a 2D array of thousands of programmable micro-machined sensors which essentially perform the same function as the piezoelectric transducers and offer advantages over flexibility in frequency range and ease of mass production.

The curvilinear array produces a convex beam offering a good field of vision for in-depth examination of deeper organs and is most often used in obstetrics and abdominal imaging. Typically, lower-frequency range transducers are used (2–5 MHz), enabling better penetration of the ultrasound beam. The linear array gives a rectangular beam which can offer better visualisation of more superficial structures and often operates in a higher-frequency range (7–12 MHz). The phased array uses precise control over the timing of element 'firing' which allows control of steering and focus of the ultrasound beam of triangular shape. The beam point is narrow, and the transducer has a small 'footprint' which can be useful for small acoustic windows such as the rib space when imaging the heart.

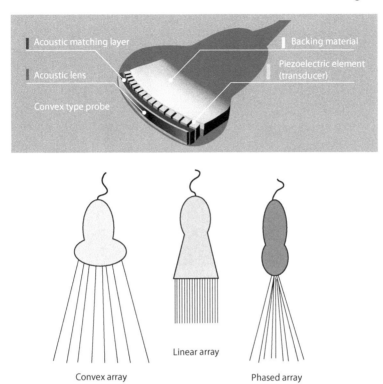

Figure 1.5 Probe construction and the commonly used probe types.

Scanning Modes

B-Mode (or Bright Modulation)

B-mode is the most common mode used to start scanning and generating a 2D grey-scale image from curvilinear, linear or phased array probes. The format of the image will depend on the probe type (see **Figure 1.6**).

M-Mode (or Motion Mode)

M-mode is a one-dimensional view along a single pre-selected line through a tissue plane. When aligned with the relevant structure it demonstrates and quantifies movement with time. This can be useful in assessing, for example, the movement of heart valves to measure incompetence or stenosis or to measure left ventricular function (see **Figure 1.7**). In the thorax it can be used to look at diaphragmatic movement and function.

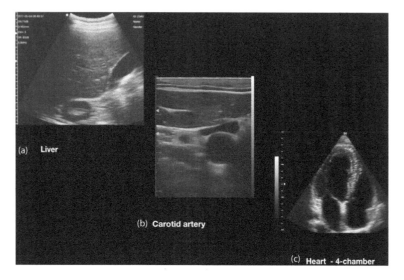

Figure 1.6 Examples of B-mode ultrasound images: (a) liver (curvilinear), (b) carotid artery (linear), (c) heart (phased array).

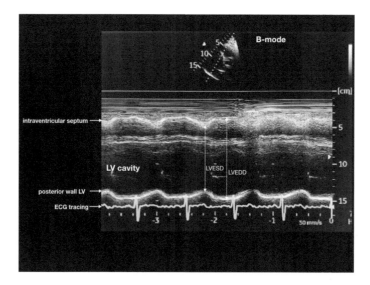

Figure 1.7 M-mode image through the heart with corresponding B-mode image above (Figure 1.6). By measuring the change in left ventricular dimensions with time throughout the cardiac cycle (this allows assessment of left ventricular function). LVEDD – left ventricular end diastolic distance, LVESD – left ventricular end systolic distance.

Colour Doppler Mode

The colour Doppler mode allows imaging of flow within the heart, arterial and venous systems within tissues. This relies on the Doppler effect to assess both the direction and velocity of flow. First described by the Austrian physicist Christian Doppler in 1842, the Doppler 'shift' is the change in frequency or wavelength of a sound wave detected at a moving observation point relative to a fixed sound wave source. The converse of this is that for a fixed observation point, a frequency shift is detected for a moving source. The commonly cited example is of the car horn which changes in pitch when approaching and then moving away from the observer. The pitch is higher than the emitted pitch when moving towards and lower when receding from the observer.

Doppler ultrasonography combines imaging of structure and function. By imaging the heart, vessel or vascular tissue, a sample volume can be positioned within a vascular structure. Powerful signal processing then calculates the phase shift over the sample volume, and both speed and direction of blood movement can be found. In the case of speed or velocity, this can be displayed as a spectral Doppler (**Figure 1.8**). Direction of flow is usually represented by a colour scale (see **Figure 1.8**) with blue indicating movement away from the transducer and red indicating movement towards the transducer. This

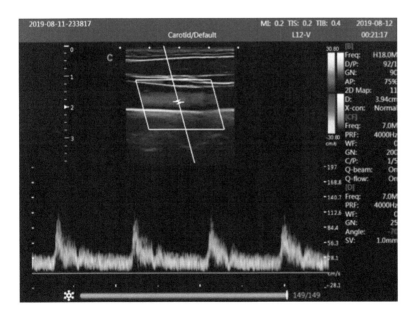

Figure 1.8 Colour Doppler image displaying colour-coded mean velocity at each point in the vessel, superimposed on B-mode image. Simultaneous display of spectral Doppler velocities measured within the sample volume located in centre of the vessel.

9

powerful physical principle can be used to quantify blood flow through heart valves and vessels which can be useful in detecting valve blockage (stenosis) or valve leakage (incompetence).

Optimising Imaging

When acquiring an ultrasound image, a number of factors must be considered before attention is given to the scanner controls in order to optimise visualisation of the relevant anatomy.

Coupling Media or Gels

The air/skin interface requires coupling media or gels to improve the acoustic contact and reduce artefact. Usually, water-soluble gels are best, as oils can dissolve rubber or plastic on transducers.

Probe Orientation

Every probe will have a notch or mark to signify the leading edge of the probe which, by convention, will correspond to the left-hand side of the screen. The convention when imaging in the longitudinal plane (see **Figure 1.9**) is that

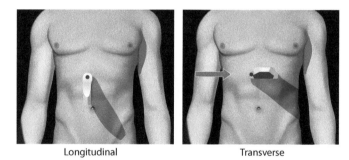

Longitudinal   Transverse

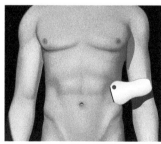

Coronal

Figure 1.9 Probe positioning and orientation conventions.

the probe should be orientated with the notch uppermost so that head to toe (craniocaudal) should be left to right on the screen. In the transverse plane the probe marker should be to the patient's right as shown, and in the coronal plane the probe marker should be uppermost as shown. In practice, an oblique plane of scanning is often used, particularly in scanning the thorax when following the rib spaces. Again, the probe marker should be kept uppermost following the same convention.

Controls and Presets

Most modern point-of-care ultrasound devices come with a wide variety of presets which can be selected depending on the anatomy to be scanned: abdominal, vascular, etc. These will reduce the need for further manual adjustment, however, inevitably factors such as body habitus and anatomical variation often require that manual adjustments be made to optimise the image. The most important variables are: frequency, gain, focus and depth (see **Figure 1.10**).

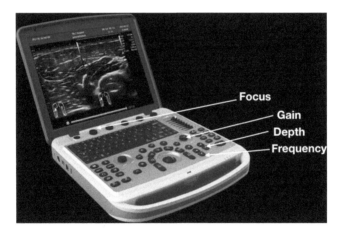

Figure 1.10 Basic controls for laptop-type ultrasound device (this image shows Sonobook range from Chison Medical Technologies). It is best to familiarise yourself with whichever ultrasound machine you have and identify the buttons prior to patient use.

Frequency

Higher frequencies mean shorter wavelengths and less tissue penetration but better spatial resolution of images, therefore, typically 10–14 MHz is a useful range for superficial vascular or musculoskeletal structures, whereas 3.5–5 MHz offers better tissue penetration for deeper structures and solid organ visualisation.

Gain

This function amplifies the ultrasound signals returning from the body. It can be thought of as a microphone function. The compromise for an amplified signal is increased noise. In obese patients, gain may need to be increased. Time gain compensation (TGC) can also be useful in compensating for the loss of intensity of signal with increasing depth. Adjustment of TGC can produce a more even grey-scale image. If increasing the gain does not provide sufficient information for diagnosis, the power of the transmitted ultrasound beam may be increased (to a maximum level) using the 'output power' control.

Focus

This can be useful in improving lateral resolution, i.e., discriminating between two structures at the same depth, and should be adjusted to the area of interest.

Depth

This function allows control over the field of vision depending on the area of interest. Ideally the whole screen should be used to optimise the view of the area of interest.

Other Functions

Even the smallest devices provide a wide range of functions, including storage of patient details, images and cine recording and calliper measurement.

Ultrasound Devices Used in Point of Care

Choosing Your Device

There is now a wide range of devices available in the POCUS market (see **Figures 1.11** and **1.12**). Choice of device will depend on a number of factors, such as cost, clinical setting, portability requirements and scanner performance. With advances in signal processing power even the smaller hand-held devices are now offering excellent image quality. The cost of POCUS has come down significantly, making the technology available to a wider range of practitioners.

Laptop Devices

A wide range of laptop devices are now available, in many cases offering increased specification over the hand-held devices. The device can be carried by hand, although if a number of probes are being used this can become unwieldy and a trolley mounted arrangement is usually preferred.

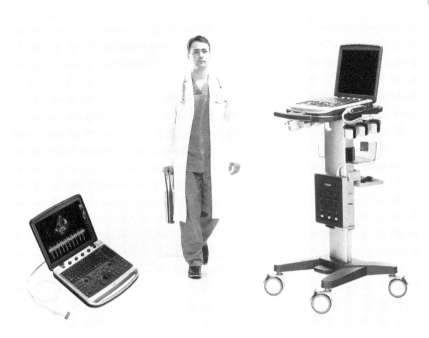

Figure 1.11 Laptop devices (Sonobook 6/8 range from Chison Medical Technologies).

Cabled

Wireless

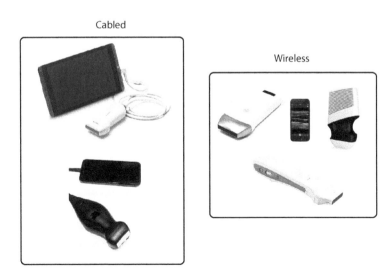

Figure 1.12 Cabled and wireless ultrasound machines.

Cabled Smartphone/Tablet Devices

A variety of cabled hand-held devices are now available that connect to purpose built screens or to mobile phones and tablet devices.

Wireless Smartphone/Tablet Devices

A wireless device offers the attraction of no cables, an enhanced ergonomic particularly around procedures. A wifi connection between a device and a smartphone/tablet ensures excellent connectivity for data exchange whilst supporting good frame rates.

Ultrasound Safety

Although ultrasound has an excellent safety record, as the ultrasound wave travels through the body, some of its energy will be deposited within the tissues through which it is travelling. Two indices have been introduced and are shown on all ultrasound scanners to provide the user with information about the potential effects which may result from the use of ultrasound. The Thermal Index (TI) provides an indication of the relative potential for a temperature rise in tissue. Three types of thermal indices may be shown: TIS (thermal index soft tissue) when insonating soft tissue; TIB (thermal index bone) when insonating near bone at focal position; and TIC (thermal index cranial) when the transducer is scanning close to bone. The Mechanical Index (MI) provides an indication of the potential of the ultrasound beam to produce a bioeffect from a non-thermal (mechanical) effect.

Clinical ultrasound should only be performed when medically indicated and undertaken by properly trained and credentialed sonographers or clinicians. The ALARA (As Low As Reasonably Achievable) principle should be adhered to. This principle refers to the use of the lowest acoustic output levels (power output) required to make an accurate sonographic diagnosis or to complete an ultrasound-guided procedure. Special care should be taken around imaging and the use of Doppler when scanning the developing foetus and during ocular applications.

Infection control measures should be adhered to according to local protocols. Generally, probes should be thoroughly cleaned between patients with non-alcohol solution. If ultrasound is being used for an invasive procedure then it should be placed within a sterile sleeve.

CHAPTER 2

POINT-OF-CARE ULTRASOUND (POCUS)

John McCafferty

Learning Objectives

- Appreciate the evolution of ultrasound over the last 60 years and how the advances in miniaturisation have led to accessible hand-held devices for POCUS.
- Understand the broad areas within the hospital setting where POCUS can be utilised.
- Have a basic knowledge of the common POCUS protocols for trauma and emergency care settings.
- Understand the utility of POCUS in the critical care setting.
- Appreciate the possibilities of POCUS in various settings (primary care, sports medicine, rural medicine, battlefield medicine, disaster/tropical medicine).
- Understand the importance of POCUS in enabling invasive procedures to be performed safely.

Ultrasound has come a long way since the pioneering work of Professor Ian Donald at the University of Glasgow in the mid-twentieth century, where early ultrasound scanners would typically occupy much of an entire room. With advances in digital technology and miniaturisation of transducers, ultrasound machines have become more and more compact and portable as clinicians rather than radiologists have come to use these devices at the bedside. The term point-of-care ultrasound (POCUS) is now well-established. The diagnostic power of ultrasound imaging has been brought to the point of care and is increasingly finding its place in a myriad of clinical settings. The use of ultrasound as a tool by the clinician is an essential skill, whether at the bedside, intensive care unit (ICU), the emergency room or outpatient clinic. Ultrasound offers a window on anatomy and complements the clinical history and physical examination to optimise rapid diagnosis and ensure safety in interventional procedures. POCUS is now beginning to be incorporated in the undergraduate training of medical students, physician assistants, advanced nurse practitioners and physiotherapists. POCUS is a rapidly evolving field with a wide variation in global uptake and many differences in practices even in healthcare systems across the developed world.

POCUS in Diagnosis

The use of POCUS in the care of hospitalised patients is extensive (**Table 2.1**), however training, uptake and provision of the technology is varied. Every hospital specialty has potential application for the use of POCUS in enhancing diagnosis, decision making and safety.

Table 2.1 Use of POCUS in Hospital/Secondary Care Settings

- Cardiac
  LV assessment, RV assessment, atrial size, pericardial effusion, chamber hypertrophy, gross valvular abnormalities
- Respiratory
  Pleural effusion, pneumothorax, consolidation, pulmonary oedema
- Abdominal/Renal
  Free fluid, gallstones, liver or splenic pathology, appendicitis, urinary retention, hydronephrosis
- Vascular
  DVT, AAA, occlusive/stenotic arterial disease, venous reflux
- Musculosceletal
  Joint effusions, fractures, active synovitis, soft tissue injuries
- Procedural
  Paracentesis, thoracocentesis, CVC placement, PIV placement, arterial line placement, arthrocentesis, abscess drainage, lumbar puncture
- Trauma
  FAST, eFAST, FEEL

Abbreviations: AAA: abdominal aortic aneurysm; CVC: central venous catheter; DVT: deep vein thrombosis; IJ: internal jugular vein; IVC: inferior vena cava; LV: left ventricle; MSK: musculoskeletal; PIV: peripheral intravenous catheter; RV: right ventricle; FAST: Focussed Assessment with Sonography for Trauma; eFAST: extended Focussed Assessment with Sonography for Trauma; FEEL: Focussed Echocardiography in Emergency Life Support.

Trauma and Emergency Care

The uptake of POCUS across the hospital specialties is still patchy, perhaps with the exception of trauma and emergency/critical care medicine. These specialties have adopted a protocol-based approach and incorporated them into curriculum requirements for training their doctors. They include the BLUE (Bedside Lung Ultrasound Emergency), RUSH (Rapid Ultrasound for Shock and Hypotension) and CLUE (Cardiovascular Limited Ultrasound Examination) protocols.

FAST Focussed Assessment with Sonography for Trauma Scan

In the UK, the best known protocol is the FAST or eFAST (extended Focussed Assessment with Sonography for Trauma, see **Table 2.2**). A trauma patient can be rapidly scanned either in the pre-hospital setting or in an accident & emergency (A&E) department (see **Figures 2.1** and **2.2**).

Table 2.2 Diagnostic Potential of eFAST Scanning

Anatomical Location	Diagnosis
Thorax	Pneumothorax
	Fractured ribs
	Haemothorax
Right flank	Intra-abdominal bleed (e.g., liver haemorrhage)
Pelvic	Intra-pelvic haematoma
Left flank	Splenic rupture/laceration and haemorrhage
Pericardial	Pericardial effusion/tamponade

FEEL (Focussed Echocardiography in Emergency Life Support)

This protocol incorporates POCUS into advanced life support (ALS) training, looking not just for potentially reversible causes of cardiac arrest but also for factors that may influence prognosis (see **Table 2.3**). Echocardiography is performed during cardiac arrest synchronised with pulse checks, thus limiting no-flow intervals during CPR (see **Figures 2.3** and **2.4**).

POCUS in Critical Care

The use of ultrasound in the critical care setting is well-established and expanding rapidly. By allowing real-time visualisation of vessels and organs it not only offers improved safety around procedures (as opposed to *blind* procedures), but it also allows enhanced real-time diagnostics in patients who are otherwise too unwell to be moved to CT or MRI scanners (see **Figure 2.5** as

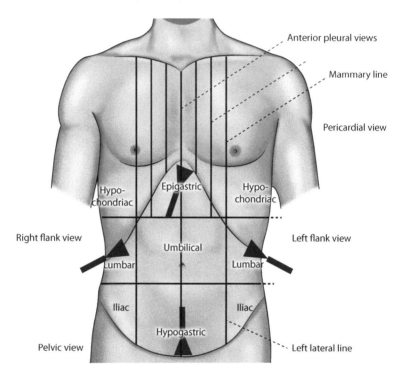

Figure 2.1 Anatomical landmarks for performing the FAST scan protocol for trauma patients.

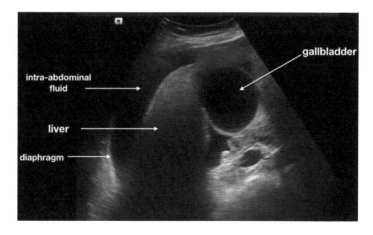

Figure 2.2 Ultrasound image from a FAST scan of right upper quadrant demonstrating intra-abdominal fluid (suggesting haemorrhage).

Table 2.3 Possible Causes for Cardiac Arrest That Could Be Identified Using POCUS

Potentially treatable causes of cardiac arrest/circulatory collapse:

- Myocardial insufficiency (including acute myocardial infarction)
- Pericardial collection (PC)
- Pulmonary embolus (PE)
- Hypovolaemia
- Tension pneumothorax

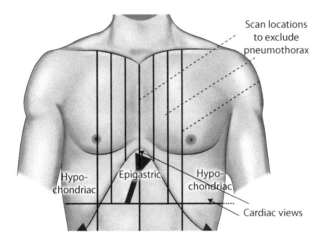

Figure 2.3 Illustrating scanning locations to identify potential reversible causes of cardiac arrest.

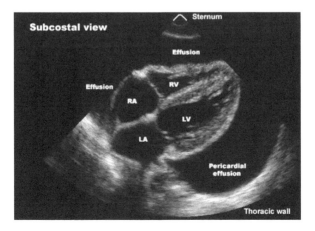

Figure 2.4 Ultrasound image from FEEL protocol demonstrating a large pericardial effusion, a potentially reversible cause of cardiac arrest.

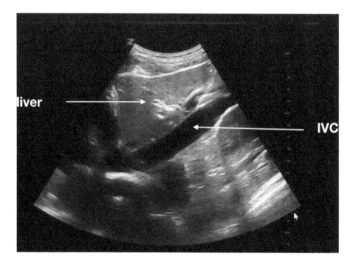

Figure 2.5 Epigastric view with ultrasound image of IVC. Evidence of respiratory collapse would indicate underfilling and requirement for further fluid resuscitation.

an example of how ultrasound can be useful in assessing critically ill patients). Table 2.4 outlines the range of uses of POCUS in the critical care setting.

Table 2.4 POCUS Use in the Critical Care Setting

Anatomical Location	Diagnosis
Thoracic	Pneumothorax in ventilated patient Pulmonary oedema Lung consolidation Pleural effusion
Cardiac (echocardiogram)	LV function Cardiac tamponade RV function
Vascular	CVC placement DVT IVC (volume status)
Abdominal/renal	Intra-abdominal collection Hydronephrosis Ascites Bladder outflow obstruction

POCUS in Primary Care

The use of POCUS in primary care will depend on healthcare settings and systems. Where primary care physicians have ready access to hospital-based ultrasound services there will be less incentive for POCUS to be widely adopted by general practitioners (GPs). Globally, however, in settings with poor access due to rurality or resource limitations there is increased uptake of POCUS by primary care providers. Studies from the United States healthcare system show good evidence of POCUS as a screening tool for heart failure, abdominal aortic aneurysm (AAA), gallstones and deep vein thrombosis (DVT). A number of primary care physicians in the UK and Europe are finding POCUS useful in these areas, as well as for diagnosing musculoskeletal injuries or directing intra-articular steroid injections. As training and technology become more readily available it is expected that we will see a growing uptake of POCUS in primary care.

Sports Medicine

Within sports medicine, POCUS is proving to be an increasingly useful tool for medics and physiotherapists where it is not only used in the diagnostics of acute injuries but also in assessing chronic injuries and monitoring response to treatment. Additionally, due to its portability, POCUS can be used on the playing field for rapid on-the-spot diagnosis (see **Figure 2.6**).

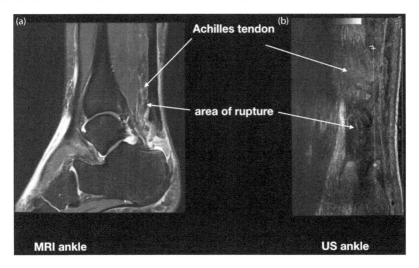

Figure 2.6 Example of Achilles tendon tear in footballer.

POCUS for Safety in Image-Guided Procedures

The majority of invasive procedures were performed up until the last decade often only using anatomical landmarks as a guide (*blind*). This has been demonstrated to be an unreliable and potentially unsafe way to carry out invasive procedures. Ultrasound offers a window on anatomy so that with the appropriate training an operator can precisely image the relevant anatomical structures and thereby ensure a safe and precise procedure. With an increased awareness of safety, ultrasound is increasingly becoming mandatory for invasive procedures and becoming embedded in clinical guidelines.

Vascular Access

Vascular access is a common invasive procedure which hospital patients undergo. This may be a peripheral venous cannula, a midline or a peripherally inserted central catheter (PICC line) placement if more prolonged venous access is required (see **Figure 2.7**). In the critical care setting, a central venous line placement is often required.

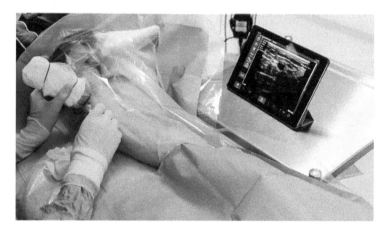

Figure 2.7 Injecting local anaesthetic above the basilic vein using wireless ultrasound (in preparation for either midline or PICC line placement).

Pleural/Ascitic Drainage

The presence of fluid in the pleural cavity (pleural effusion) or within the abdomen (ascites) often requires drainage, either for symptom relief or to obtain fluid samples to aid diagnosis. The placement of a drainage catheter can be potentially dangerous, risking the inadvertent puncture of a vascular structure or other organ. POCUS aids accurate placement of the catheter into the collection of fluid (see **Figure 2.8**).

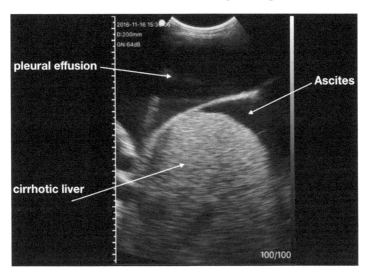

Figure 2.8 Large right pleural effusion in patient with cirrhosis and ascites.

Nerve Blocks

Nerve blocks are carried out in a number of settings in order to achieve regional anaesthesia most often in the surgical setting. In **Figure 2.9**, a tibial

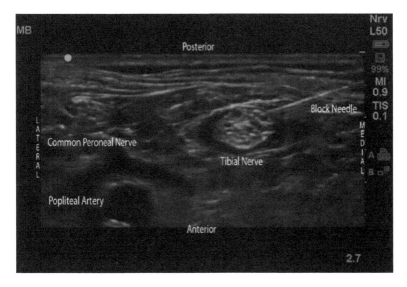

Figure 2.9 Tibial nerve block in a patient with a deep laceration to the sole of foot requiring wound exploration.

nerve block is carried out under ultrasound guidance to anaesthetise the foot below the level of the ankle prior to surgery. Ultrasound guidance improves efficacy of nerve blocks and minimises the risk of complications.

Joint Aspiration

Joint effusions often require intervention to exclude septic arthritis and aid diagnosis in the acutely swollen joint. Ultrasound ensures accurate needle placement, avoiding vessels and nerves to ensure a safe arthrocentesis (see **Figure 2.10**).

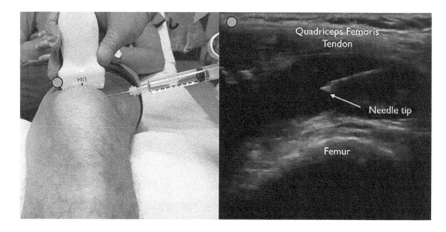

Figure 2.10 Aspiration of the right knee in a pyrexial patient with an acutely swollen joint.

PART II
ULTRASOUND ASSESSMENTS BY BODY SYSTEM

CHAPTER 3

NECK ULTRASOUND

Kirsten MS Kind

Learning Objectives

- Have a knowledge of the anatomy of the neck, including the thyroid, parathyroid and salivary glands; carotid and major vessels and lymph node groups.
- Understand your choice of ultrasound probe when imaging the neck.
- Be able to carry out a basic ultrasound assessment of the neck and identify the normal anatomical structures.
- Have a basic understanding of common pathologies of the neck that can be diagnosed using ultrasound.

Anatomy of the Neck

The anatomy of the neck can be complex and can be studied to almost infinite depth. In this chapter, we hope to give a general overview of the relevant anatomy as it applies to the practitioner as they commence and expand their ultrasound practice.

Thyroid Gland

The thyroid gland lies anterior to the thyroid and cricoid cartilages of the larynx and extends from the level of the fifth cervical vertebra (C5) down to the first thoracic vertebra (T1). It has two lobes, one on either side of the trachea, which are joined in the midline by the isthmus. Each lobe has a superior and inferior pole. The arterial supply comes from the superior and inferior thyroid arteries, with venous drainage via the superior, middle and inferior thyroid veins (see **Figure 3.1**).

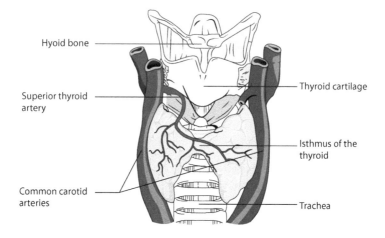

Figure 3.1 Regional anatomy of the thyroid gland.

Parathyroid Glands

There are usually four (sometimes up to twelve) parathyroid glands which lie posterior to the thyroid gland. The superior pair usually lie posterior to the middle third of the thyroid, with the inferior pair of parathyroid glands lateral to the inferior pole of the thyroid. These glands are small, ovoid and, unless pathologically enlarged, difficult to see on ultrasound.

Salivary Glands

There are two main groups of salivary glands that we commonly evaluate on ultrasound: the parotid and submandibular glands (see **Figure 3.2**). The sublingual glands are difficult to evaluate on ultrasound thanks to their small size and location under the tongue. The parotid glands lie just anterior to the ear (in the parotid space) and can extend as far down as the angle of the jaw. They wrap around the rami of the mandible and have both deep and superficial lobes. The facial nerve passes through the parotid gland, as do the external carotid artery and retromandibular vein. It is common to encounter small lymph nodes within the parotid glands, which are considered a normal variant. The submandibular glands are situated behind the mandible on both sides of the face. They have deep and superficial lobes and excrete saliva into the floor of the mouth via the submandibular ducts.

Vessels

Several important vascular structures travel through the neck, and ultrasound is an excellent way to evaluate these vessels. The main artery is the carotid,

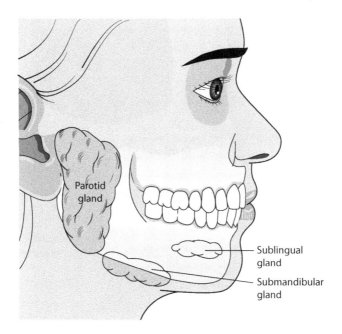

Figure 3.2 Illustration of the anatomy of salivary glands.

which divides into the internal and external carotid arteries mid-way up the neck at the approximate level of the thyroid cartilage. Lateral to the carotid arteries on both sides of the neck are the internal jugular veins. The smaller external jugular veins pass superficially over the sternocleidomastoid muscles and are of less clinical significance (see **Figure 3.3**).

Lymph Nodes

There are several important groups of lymph nodes in the neck, and ultrasound is an excellent tool for evaluating them. They can be grouped by anatomical location or by level – the former is more often used on clinical examination, while the latter is often used by oncologists and radiologists (see **Figure 3.4**).

Lymph nodes, wherever they are located, should be of similar morphology. They should be roughly ovoid in shape, with a clear fatty hilum and otherwise uniform echogenicity. If a node is enlarged, but maintains this normal morphology, it is more likely to be a reactive node than a malignant node. Any node which measures greater than 1 cm in short axis is considered 'enlarged.' If a node demonstrates mixed echogenicity, has lost its fatty hilum and/or has become rounded in shape, it is suspicious for malignant infiltration and should be investigated with further imaging or biopsy/resection. Abnormal nodes

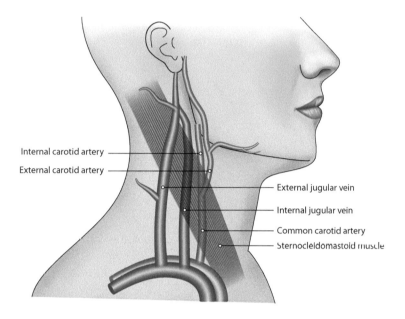

Figure 3.3 Demonstrating the major vasculature of the neck.

may also merge together to form a larger, lobulated nodal mass, while normal or simple enlarged nodes tend to 'cluster' rather than merge.

Ultrasound Imaging of Thyroid

Technique

Using a high-frequency, linear array probe, begin in the transverse plane, in the midline. Sweep through the whole gland in this plane and save images of the isthmus and each lobe. Rotate the probe by 90° and interrogate each lobe of thyroid individually, saving further images in this plane. The whole gland should be uniform in texture, with each lobe being roughly the same size. If a focal nodule is identified, obtaining images in two different planes with maximum dimensions and colour Doppler is essential. See **Figure 3.5** to visualise a normal thyroid gland.

Pathology

Diseases affecting the thyroid gland can be divided into two categories: diffuse and focal. Diffuse thyroid pathologies (Graves' disease, Hashimoto's thyroiditis) tend to cause diffuse enlargement of the thyroid gland, with

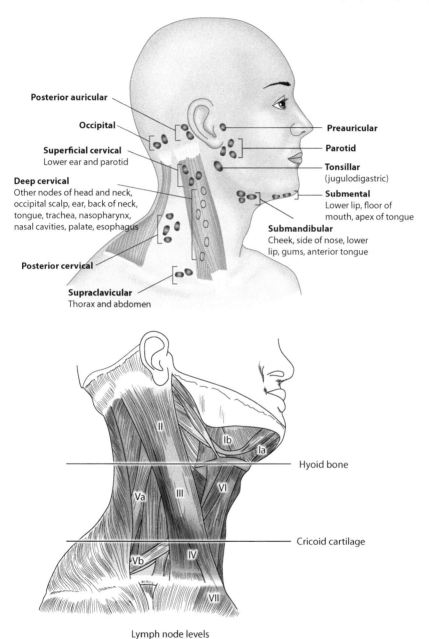

Figure 3.4 Anatomical groups and lymph node levels in the neck.

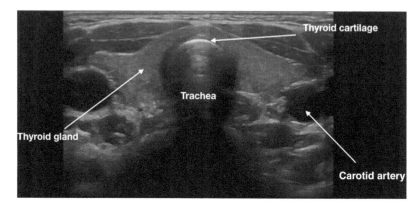

Figure 3.5 Ultrasound image of normal thyroid gland and adjacent anatomical structures.

heterogenous echotexture. They may or may not have focal nodules as well. Focal thyroid nodules can be further divided into benign or malignant nodules. Though we can never be 100% sure whether a lesion is malignant on ultrasound, there are several features that we can specifically look for and document to help raise or lower suspicion and trigger further investigation.

Features suspicious of malignancy:

- Irregular margins
- Longer (craniocaudally) than wide (transverse)
- Intranodular flow on colour Doppler
- Hypoechoic
- Calcifications

Almost all of these features can also be found in benign nodules, although each favours malignancy to a greater or lesser extent. Most lesions exhibiting one of these features will undergo further investigation and, if more than one feature is present, biopsy or fine needle aspiration (FNA) is indicated. A scoring system is available from the American College of Radiology (ACR) for assessing thyroid lesions on ultrasound to aid management decisions regarding follow-up and further imaging/investigation. This is called the Thyroid Imaging Reporting and Data System (TI-RADS) and is easily accessible on the Internet.

Ultrasound Imaging of Salivary Glands

Technique

Images should be obtained in two orthogonal planes of each major salivary gland (parotid, submandibular and sublingual if visible) with images of both

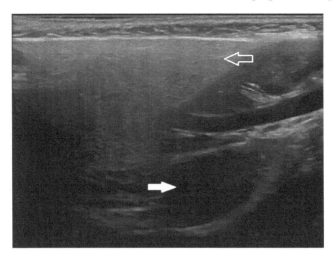

Figure 3.6 Ultrasound image of the parotid gland. The hollow white arrow is the parotid gland in longitudinal section, and the solid white arrow is the jugular vein.

sides regardless of site of concern. Again, a high-frequency, linear array is the most appropriate probe for imaging the neck as most structures are superficial. See **Figure 3.6** for an ultrasound image of a normal parotid gland.

Pathology

Diffuse enlargement of a salivary gland can have a number of causes and can be difficult to appreciate. For this reason, splitting your screen and having images of each paired gland side by side can be extremely helpful for picking up subtle-sized discrepancies or differences in echotexture. Focal salivary gland lesions, like thyroid nodules, should be measured in two planes and be interrogated with colour Doppler. The majority of focal salivary gland lesions are benign; however, most will require biopsy for certainty so thorough evaluation on ultrasound is essential for further decision making. Unfortunately, criteria for delineating between benign and malignant lesions are less well-defined in the salivary glands, so we are usually unable to say one way or the other on ultrasound. Location may be helpful. Lesions within the sublingual gland are more likely to be malignant than those in the submandibular glands which are, in turn, more likely to be malignant than parotid gland lesions. It is normal to see small lymph nodes within the salivary glands. They should be small, well-circumscribed and clearly have normal lymph node morphology. Enlarged nodes or nodes demonstrating any abnormal features should raise concern.

Ultrasound Imaging of Vessels of the Neck

A high-frequency, linear array probe with a wide footprint is a good choice for imaging the neck vessels, to allow more of the vessel to fit on the screen. As a beginner it is important to be able to identify the following major vascular structures in the neck:

- Common carotid artery (CCA)
- Internal/external carotid arteries (ICA/ECA)
- Internal jugular vein (IJV)

In a healthy normal patient, the arteries should be seen to be pulsating with no gross evidence of disease (i.e., plaque/ulceration) within the vessels. Similarly, the internal jugular vein should be identifiable as a larger structure lying adjacent to the carotid artery that is easily compressible (see **Figure 3.7**). Vascular scanning is explored in further detail in Chapters 8 and 9, and as per these chapters colour Doppler/pulse wave Doppler can be used to explore these vessels in further detail. However, it is important to recognise that neck vascular scanning, specifically carotid/vertebral artery scanning, is a highly-specialised area. If the scanning is performed by a beginner and if any area of abnormality is identified, the patient should be referred to a dedicated vascular sonographer for a more detailed scan.

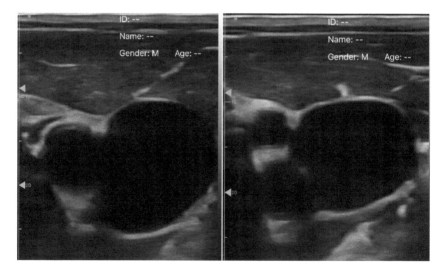

Figure 3.7 Major vessels of the neck. The image on the left shows the smaller common carotid artery lying adjacent to the larger internal jugular vein. The image on the right (when moving further up the neck with the ultrasound probe) shows the common carotid splitting into the internal and external carotid arteries.

Ultrasound Imaging of Lymph Nodes

Technique

As with other structures in the neck, a high-frequency, linear probe will give detailed images of superficial nodes (see **Figure 3.8**). A structured approach to the nodal stations is helpful. Direct comparison with the contralateral side can be really useful when trying to distinguish normal from abnormal nodes.

Pathology

Abnormal lymph nodes can have a number of causes, usually secondary to either infection or malignancy. The presenting history will give the practitioner clues as to which is the most likely diagnosis in the patient.

Features of concern for malignancy in a node:

- Rounded, rather than ovoid shape
- Loss of normal fatty hilum
- Increased vascularity
- Heterogenous echotexture
- Areas of internal necrosis
- Large (>1 cm short axis)
- Clumping of several nodes together

Children are often referred for ultrasound of the neck because of a palpable lump, usually felt by parents. These lumps often correspond to morphologically normal lymph nodes which can be nicely demonstrated on ultrasound and confidently dismissed by experienced paediatric sonographers.

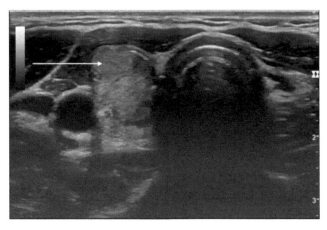

Figure 3.8 Normal level II lymph nodes in the neck of a 7 year old. Note the hypoechoic fatty hilum (arrow). They each measure less than 1 cm in short axis.

Examples of Common Pathology (Figures 3.9–3.12)

Thyroid Tumour

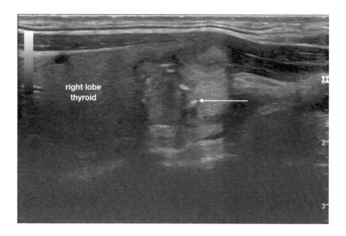

Figure 3.9 Mixed echogenicity lesion in the right lobe of the thyroid (white arrow).

Thyroglossal Duct Cyst

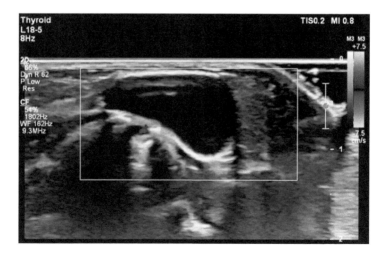

Figure 3.10 Thyroglossal duct cyst. Note the simple appearance with homogenous hypoechogenicity internally and lack of any Doppler signal.

Lymphoma

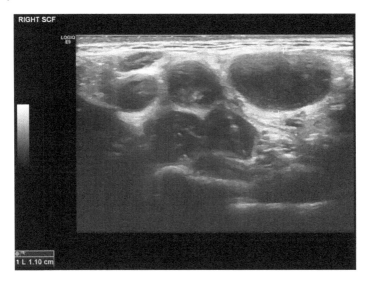

Figure 3.11 Multiple abnormal lymph nodes due to lymphoma.

Parotid Gland Lipoma

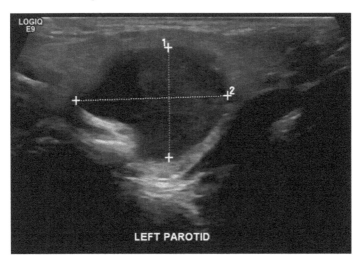

Figure 3.12 Lipoma of the parotid gland. Note the normal, homogenously hyperechoic parotid gland at the top of the image. This lesion was indeterminate on ultrasound and went onto biopsy which found it to be a benign lipoma.

CHAPTER 4

THORACIC ULTRASOUND

John McCafferty

Learning Objectives

- Gain an understanding of basic thoracic anatomy relevant to ultrasound examination of the thorax.
- Appreciate the context of an ultrasound examination in making a diagnosis.
- Be able to carry out an ultrasound examination of the thorax following a systematic approach.
- Acquire and interpret ultrasound images of the thorax in a normal healthy subject.
- Additionally, be able to recognise the common pathological respiratory conditions that can be diagnosed with ultrasound.

Point-of-care ultrasound (POCUS) of the thorax should be carried out wherever possible in association with a full respiratory history and clinical examination, along with knowledge of the patient's relevant blood results. POCUS in many cases will help to discriminate between your differential diagnoses and allow you to arrive at a robust diagnosis with confidence. It can also help determine the need for other relevant investigations such as chest radiography, CT/MRI scanning, cardiac echo, etc. The ability to accurately define thoracic anatomy will also allow you to carry out procedures such as pleural aspiration and chest drain placement safely.

Thoracic Anatomy

The thorax presents a particular challenge to imaging with ultrasound. Firstly, it is surrounded by a bony ribcage so acoustic windows are limited to the intercostal spaces (see **Figure 4.1**). Secondly, the lungs are air-filled structures and thus strongly reflect the ultrasound. However, the boundaries of the thorax can be defined using the appropriate landmarks: the right

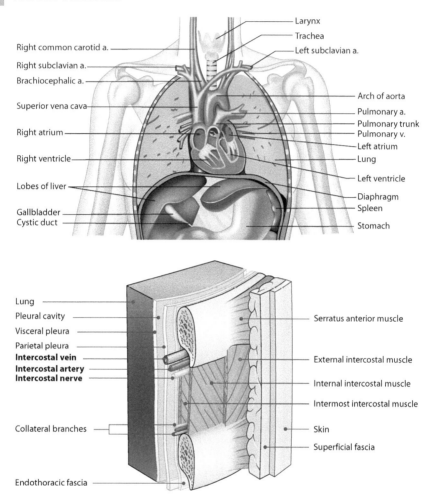

Figure 4.1 Thoracic anatomy including detail of the intercostal space.

hemidiaphragm and liver, the left hemidiaphragm and spleen inferiorly. The pleura can be seen anteriorly, laterally and superiorly by careful examination through the intercostal spaces in these areas.

Ultrasound Features of Thoracic Anatomy

The Intercostal View

Figure 4.2 illustrates the ultrasound image through the intercostal space. Starting superficially, identify the subcutaneous tissue and fat, then the

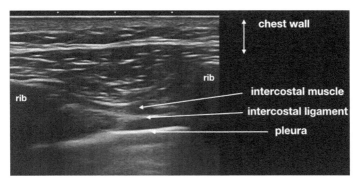

Figure 4.2 Intercostal space highlighting rib shadows, pleural line and A-lines.

intercostal muscle, distinct for its striated appearance and fascial planes. The space is bounded by the bright or high attenuating bony rib with acoustic shadow extending deep to the rib. The bright or echogenic pleural line is seen deep to the muscle. With higher resolution (frequency) probes the visceral and parietal pleural surfaces can also be identified. Observe these lines gliding during respiration – the so-called 'gliding sign' or 'sliding sign.' Deep to the pleura is the air-filled lung which appears dark with faint reverberation artefact from the pleura – these transverse lines are termed A-lines.

Right Inferior/Liver Window

Define the right inferior border of the thorax with the probe positioned at the level of the eighth intercostal space on the mid-axillary line (see **Figure 4.3**).

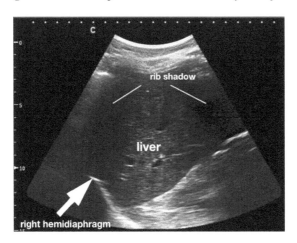

Figure 4.3 US image demonstrating right costophrenic angle with the liver and right hemidiaphragm.

Left Inferior/Splenic Window

On the left, at the level of the eighth intercostal space on the mid-axillary line, define the left inferior border of the thorax, identifying the left hemidiaphragm with the spleen below (see **Figure 4.4**).

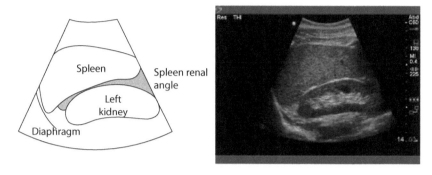

Figure 4.4 US image demonstrating left costophrenic angle with the spleen and left hemidiaphragm.

Basic Thoracic Ultrasound Assessment

Preparation

In preparation for an ultrasound exam the practitioner must have a clear understanding of the clinical indication for the examination, any associated procedures and the clinical questions the examination seeks to address. This must then be explained to the patient prior to obtaining verbal or in some cases written consent to proceed with the examination. A 3.5–5 MHz curvilinear array probe offers the optimum frequency range in order to visualise the pleura, lung and diaphragm, along with the solid organs which border the thorax inferiorly. Generally, the abdominal preset is a good starting point but depending on the exam subject be prepared to adjust settings to optimise your image as outlined in Chapter 1.

- Introduce yourself to the patient.
- Explain the procedure and gain verbal consent.
- Wash your hands and put on gloves.
- Ensure the probe has been cleaned with an alcohol wipe.
- Have a chaperone present throughout your assessment.
- Have the patient dressed in an examination gown to allow exposure of the chest during examination.
- Position the patient seated on an examination couch at 45° (see **Figure 4.5**).

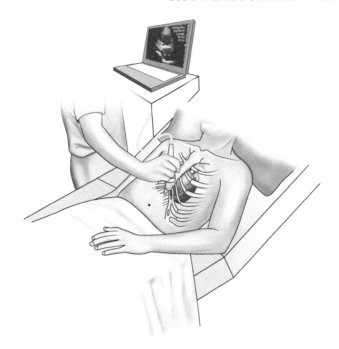

Figure 4.5 Positioning of patient for ultrasound examination of the thorax.

Image Acquisition

The following outlines a systematic ultrasound examination of the thorax excluding cardiac assessment which will be covered in Chapter 5. In clinical practice this may be modified according to the clinical scenario. See **Figure 4.6** to appreciate the relevant chest surface anatomy to guide your ultrasound examination.

- With the subject comfortably sitting at 45°, start by examining the anterior chest. Apply the ultrasound probe with the leading edge uppermost starting with the second intercostal space on the left observing the ultrasound image to identify the echogenic pleural line and the 'sliding sign' with respiration.
- Alternating between left and right sides continue your examination down to the eighth intercostal space. At each location appreciate the anatomy of the intercostal space and lung.
- At the eighth intercostal space move laterally into the anterior axillary line to define the liver and right hemidiaphragm on the right and on the left the spleen and left hemidiaphragm.

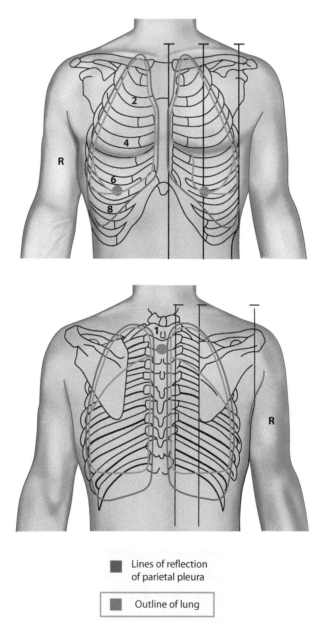

Lines of reflection
of parietal pleura

Outline of lung

Figure 4.6 Illustrating the chest surface markings to guide the ultrasound examination.

- In each case move more laterally into the mid-axillary line to further define the lower border of the thorax together with confirmation of diaphragmatic movement with respiration.
- Next, sit the patient forward and repeat the procedure to examine the posterior chest.

Closing Steps

- Make sure you have recorded your findings and saved any relevant images.
- Thank the patient.
- Wipe off the ultrasound gel from the patient's skin.
- If appropriate, help patient to dress.
- Discuss your clinical and ultrasound examination findings with the patient.
- Decide upon further investigations/treatment as necessary.

Common Respiratory Pathologies

Having familiarised yourself with the ultrasound appearances of normal thoracic anatomy, we now will consider some common pathological findings commonly that are encountered in the routine clinical setting.

Pleural Effusion

A pleural effusion describes the abnormal accumulation of fluid in the pleural space. This can be due to a wide variety of causes. They are often grouped into 'transudative' or 'exudative' causes depending on their protein content and other factors. A wide differential often requires both visualisation of the effusion using ultrasound and safe sampling of the fluid under ultrasound guidance.

CASE EXAMPLE 1

A 65-year-old man presents with progressive breathlessness and weight loss. He is an ex-smoker and previously worked as a joiner where he was exposed to asbestos. On examination he appears of low BMI, is comfortable at rest with oxygen saturations of 96% on room air, with a normal pulse and blood pressure. His heart sounds are normal with no murmurs on chest auscultation. Examination of the chest reveals reduced expansion on the right with a stony dull percussion note and absent breath sounds.

His blood panel is unremarkable, but his chest radiograph and ultrasound are shown in **Figure 4.7**.

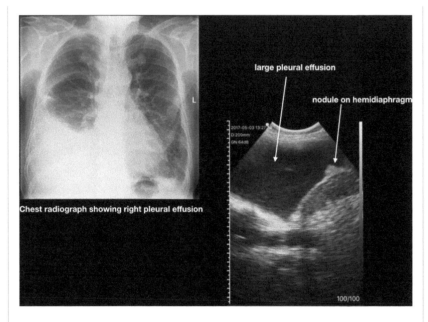

Figure 4.7 Large right pleural effusion seen on chest radiograph (left image). Ultrasound (right image) appearance confirms the presence of a large unilateral pleural effusion with nodularity on the right hemidiaphragm.

Consolidated Lung (Pneumonia)

Pneumonia can be caused by a bacterial or viral infection of the lung and can cause significant morbidity and mortality. The body's inflammatory response results in the efflux of inflammatory cells and fluid replacing a region of lung resulting in a process termed 'consolidation.'

CASE EXAMPLE 2

A 39-year-old female presents with a 5-day history of fever, cough and left-sided pleuritic chest pain. Her past medical history is unremarkable. On examination she appears flushed and is in obvious discomfort. Oxygen saturations are 92% on room air. The rest of her observations reveal a temperature of 39°C, pulse 120/min and BP 90/40 mmHg. Examination of her chest demonstrates a dull percussion note on the left with diminished breath sounds. Her blood results reveal a significant neutrophilia and a C-reactive protein (CRP) of 200.

Her chest radiograph and ultrasound are shown in **Figure 4.8**.

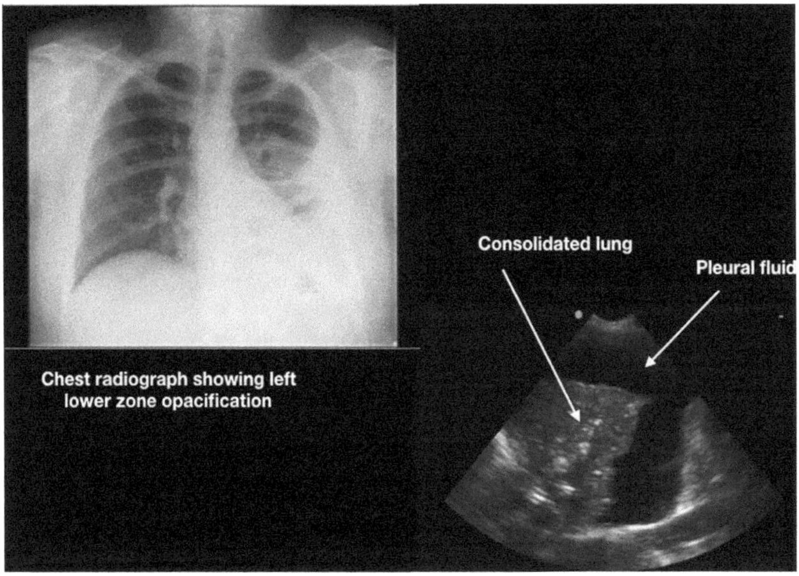

Consolidated lung

Pleural fluid

Chest radiograph showing left
lower zone opacification

Figure 4.8 Chest radiograph (left) shows a raised left hemidiaphragm and opacification of the left mid- and lower zones of her lungs. The ultrasound (left) confirmed the high position of the left hemidiaphragm with the presence of a moderate left pleural effusion and a densely consolidated underlying lung.

Pneumothorax

A pneumothorax occurs when there is a breach within the visceral pleura allowing air to escape from the underlying lung into the pleural space.

CASE EXAMPLE 3

A 16-year-old male presents with sudden onset of right-sided chest discomfort and breathlessness. He is a smoker but has an unremarkable past medical history. On examination, he has a tall, slim build and his oxygen saturations are 94% on room air. He has reduced expansion on the right side with a hyper-resonant percussion note and poorly audible breath sounds on the right.

His chest radiograph and ultrasound are shown in **Figure 4.9**.

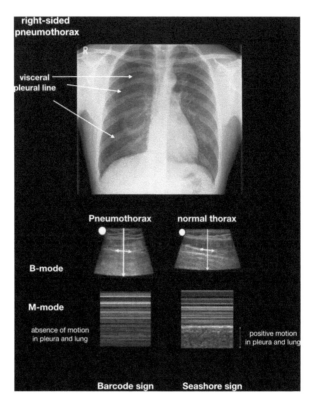

Figure 4.9 Chest radiograph (upper image) shows large right-sided pneumothorax. Lower image shows ultrasound image in both B-mode and M-mode of pneumothorax and normal side of thorax. With the pneumothorax the pleural 'sliding sign is absent and in M-mode no pleural or lung motion is seen which creates a series of static horizontal lines giving the overall appearance of a 'barcode'. This is in contrast to the normal side where pleural and lung motion is detected as a blurred image creating an overall image akin to a 'seashore'.

Pulmonary Oedema

Pulmonary oedema describes the accumulation of fluid within the lung interstitial and alveolar space usually as a result of acute heart failure.

CASE EXAMPLE 4

A 65-year-old female presents with an acute onset of breathlessness and difficulty lying flat. She has a past history of ischaemic heart disease and is known to have impairment of left ventricular function. On attendance in A&E she is tachypnoeic with a raised jugular venous pressure, and she has significant ankle oedema. Her oxygen saturations are 89% on room air, heart rate is 105 and blood pressure is 90/60 mmHg. On auscultation of both her lung fields you identify reduced air entry bibasally with coarse crepitations throughout.

Her chest radiograph and ultrasound are shown in **Figure 4.10**.

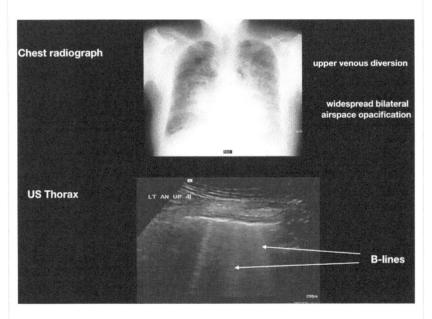

Figure 4.10 Chest radiograph demonstrating features of pulmonary oedema with widespread bilateral alveolar shadowing and upper lobe venous diversion. The corresponding ultrasound image demonstrates the presence of B-lines which are seen as vertical lines radiating deep into the lung from the pleural surface. B-lines correspond to the thickening of subpleural interlobular septa in pulmonary oedema and are sometimes also seen due to fibrotic thickening in pulmonary fibrosis.

CHAPTER 5

CARDIAC ULTRASOUND

Nick B Spath, Anoop SV Shah and Shirjel R Alam

Learning Objectives

- Understand cardiac anatomy relevant for echocardiographic assessment.
- Appreciate the technique for acquiring echocardiographic views of the heart.
- Understand how best to optimise and interpret echocardiographic images.
- Be able to recognise normal cardiac morphology using ultrasound.
- Be able to recognise key cardiac abnormalities using ultrasound.

Introduction

This chapter gives an overview of cardiac anatomy and pathology that can be seen using point-of-care ultrasound assessment of the heart. The technique for acquiring echocardiographic windows is of paramount importance as this determines the quality and utility of the cardiac assessment. In this chapter, eight standard windows are discussed in detail, and we aim to provide techniques and tips on how best to acquire, optimise and interpret echocardiographic images. In clinical practice, perhaps the most common indication for point-of-care cardiac echocardiographic assessment is to gauge left ventricular systolic function. However, many additional cardiac structures can easily be interrogated by an operator with the right skills. The aim is to visualise as much cardiac anatomy as possible with as much accuracy and detail as possible, in order to draw clinically relevant conclusions. With this in mind, we next discuss the structure and function of key cardiac structures in turn: the left and right ventricles, the atria, the valves and pericardial/intra-cardiac structures, covering key pathologies of interest which are relevant to point-of-care echocardiography assessment. Colour Doppler is a useful additional tool to visually appreciate pathological blood flow within and around the cardiac structures and is applied in point-of-care echocardiography as a qualitative tool which points to the need for further assessment. More in-depth discussion of ultrasound physics and quantitative Doppler assessment of the heart is beyond the scope of this chapter, and is discussed in detail elsewhere. The normal ranges quoted here are based on the American Society of Echocardiography Guidelines, 2015.

Image Acquisition

Typically, cardiac imaging requires the use of intercostal acoustic windows, necessitating the use of ultrasound probes with a smaller area and a frequency range from 2 MHz to 7.5 MHz. Cardiac imaging in adults requires the use of lower frequencies (typically 2–4 MHz). Generally speaking, the patient is ideally placed in a left lateral position, with operators conventionally sitting at the patient's right-hand side. From here, the operator holds the probe in their right hand, reaching across the patient to acquire images, with the echocardiography machine in-front and to their left (see **Figures 5.1** and **5.2**). Some operators adapt their technique to use alternative positions, but this is an individual choice. The probe has a marker on one side, corresponding to an equivalent marker on the image, enabling orientation.

Parasternal Long Axis

For the parasternal long-axis view, the marker of the transducer points somewhat towards the right shoulder (see **Figures 5.3** and **5.4**). The optimal window will vary according to individual patient body habitus.

In this view, the apex should not usually be visible, but the posterior and septal regional walls of the left ventricle can be seen, allowing a good initial assessment of overall left ventricular function as well as the motion of the interventricular septum. Visual assessment of the left atrium and left-sided valves may also be made, with regurgitation often visible with colour Doppler. The size of the aortic root can also be assessed here and occasionally an aortic dissection may be seen in this view. Whilst the right ventricle is not well-visualised in this view, an anterior or posterior pericardial effusion may be seen.

Parasternal Short Axis

Keeping the probe at the same position but rotating 90° clockwise will obtain a parasternal short-axis (PSAX) view. By tilting the transducer between superior, neutral and inferior angulations, views of the aortic valve, mitral valve and mid-left ventricular views are obtained (see **Figures 5.5** and **5.6**).

As well as visualising aortic and mitral valve apparatus, these short-axis views are a good opportunity to assess left ventricular systolic function, particularly when identifying regional wall motion abnormalities.

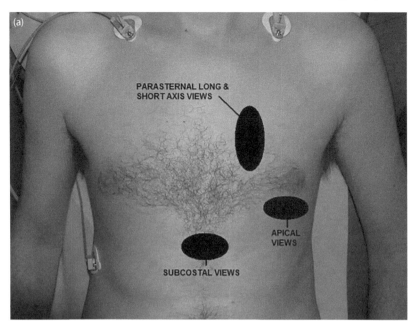

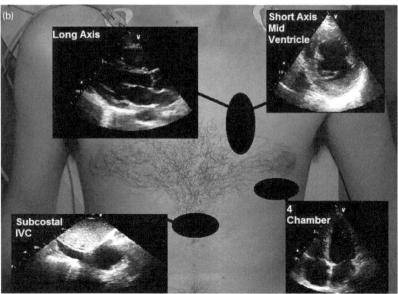

Figure 5.1 (a) Key probe positions to conduct a standard transthoracic echocardiographic study. (b) Corresponding 2-dimensional echocardiographic images obtained from each of these positions.

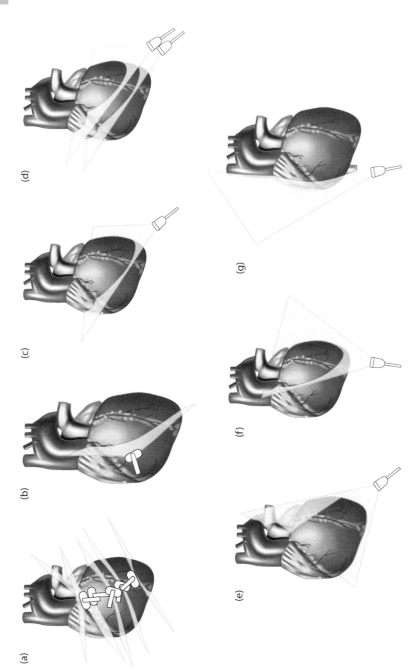

Figure 5.2 Diagrammatic representation of all six views obtained from the three echocardiography windows. (a) and (b) Parasternal short-axis and long-axis, (c) apical 4-chamber, (d) LV outflow tract, (e) apical 2-chamber, (f) and (g) subcostal views.

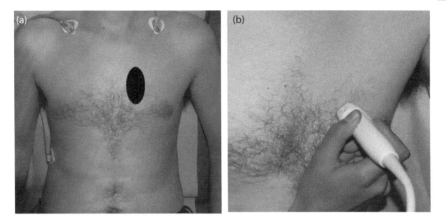

Figure 5.3 Position of the probe for the parasternal long-axis view.

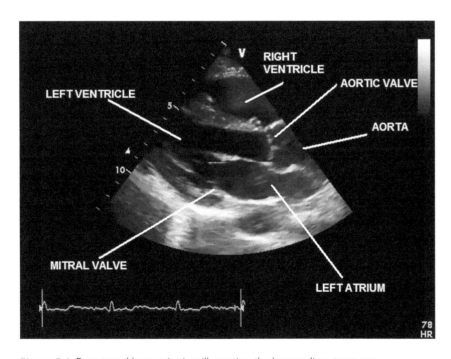

Figure 5.4 Parasternal long-axis view illustrating the key cardiac structures.

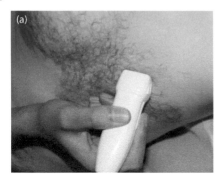
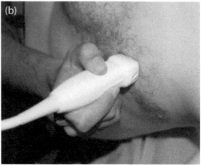
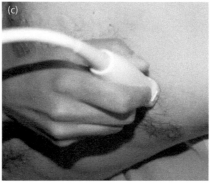

Figure 5.5 Position of the probe for the parasternal short-axis view.

Apical Views

This is a very versatile imaging window, allowing assessment of the left ventricle in the long-axis orientation, starting with the probe at the apex which is usually at the fifth intercostal space. Begin with the apical 4-chamber view, where the marker on the probe should be pointed towards the patient's left shoulder. In this view, all four chambers of the heart are well-visualised, allowing further assessment of regional wall motion of the inferoseptum and anterolateral walls. Colour Doppler further aids in the interrogation of the atrioventricular valves. Take care that you are imaging the true apex and are not too superior, which can foreshorten the view and misrepresent function, seen when the apex appears to contract (see **Figure 5.7**).

From this position, rotate the transducer approximately 60° anti-clockwise to result in a 2-chamber long-axis view. This enables assessment of the true inferior and anterior walls, as well as further views of the left atrium and mitral valve (see **Figure 5.8**).

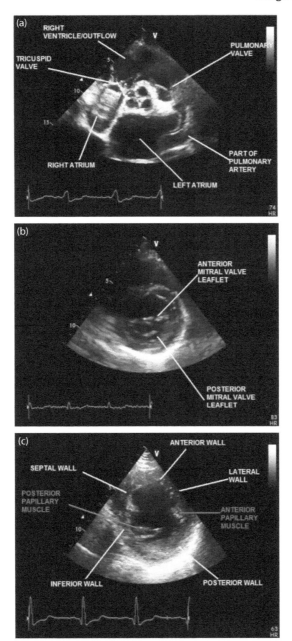

Figure 5.6 Parasternal short-axis views at the level of the aortic valve (a), mitral valve (b) and papillary muscle (c).

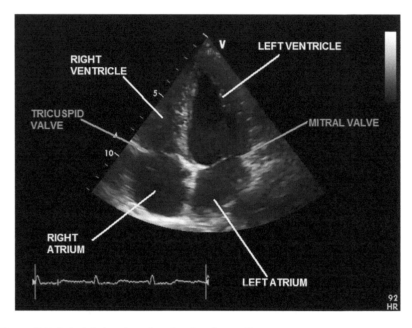

Figure 5.7 Apical 4-chamber view showing the cardiac structures.

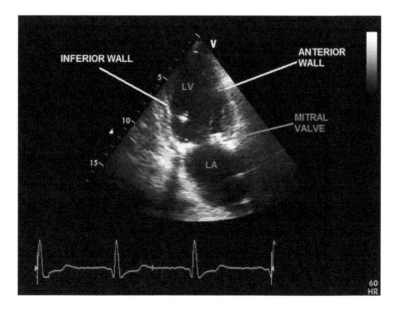

Figure 5.8 Apical 2-chamber view showing the cardiac structures.

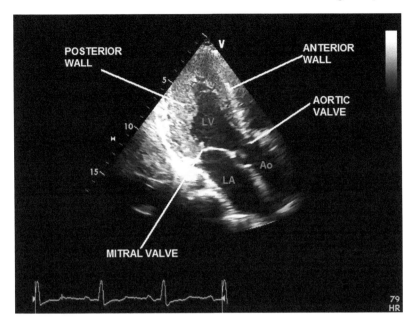

Figure 5.9 Apical 3-chamber view showing the cardiac structures.

Rotating the transducer anti-clockwise by another 60° brings a 3-chamber image into view, also known as the apical long-axis 3-chamber view. This view provides functional assessment of the anteroseptum and inferolateral left ventricular walls, as well as demonstrating the left ventricular outflow tract, aortic valve and mitral valve (see **Figure 5.9**).

Finally, a so-called '5-chamber' view is obtained from this apical window. Starting from the 4-chamber view, by maintaining the same rotation but tilting the probe so the beam angles superiorly, the left ventricular outflow tract and aortic valve come into view. This enables additional assessment of certain pathologies affecting these structures, particularly assessment of the aortic valve (see **Figure 5.10**).

Subcostal

Unlike the other windows discussed so far, the subcostal view is obtained with the patient lying supine, positioning the probe at the inferior border of the thoracic cage and pressing down. With the marker on the probe pointing towards the patient's left-hand side, this window will give a subcostal 4-chamber view. This appears very similar to the apical 4-chamber view, except at a slightly different angle. In addition, this window can be useful to identify pericardial collections (see **Figures 5.11** and **5.12**).

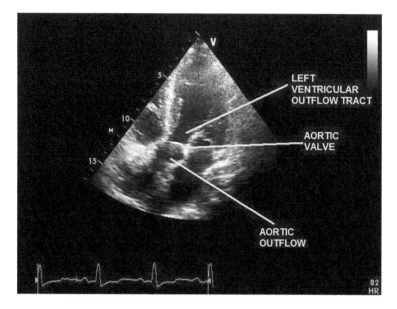

Figure 5.10 Apical 5-chamber view showing the cardiac structures.

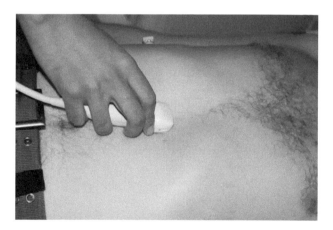

Figure 5.11 Probe position for the subcostal views.

By rotating the ultrasound probe 90° anti-clockwise, the inferior vena cava will be visible, allowing an assessment of the filling status to be made (discussed in further detail in the following sections). The subcostal view is particularly useful in emergency situations where patients may not be able to comply with positioning requests or may be ventilated where positive airway pressures make the other transthoracic windows more challenging.

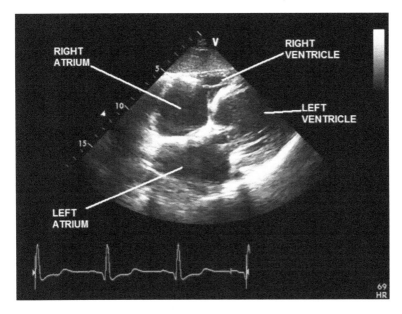

Figure 5.12 Subcostal view illustrating the key cardiac structures.

Optimising Imaging Windows

Whilst it may seem obvious, ultrasound waves travel very poorly in air and it is therefore essential that there is adequate gel to allow optimal ultrasonic conduction between the transducer and the skin. Adjustments to angulation, tilt and depth will bring the structures into the centre of the image. Increasing or decreasing the gain will allow better characterisation of valves or the endocardial border. For subcostal views, asking the patient to bend their knees to 90° and relax their abdominal muscles can significantly improve views. Finally, for transthoracic views where the quality of images can depend on movement of the lungs and thoracic cage, it may be useful to ask the patient to hold their breath in expiration.

Normal Morphology and Pathology

Cardiac Chambers

Left Ventricle

Left ventricular function is best assessed visually in the apical long-axis as well as the parasternal short-axis views. In the context of point-of-care echocardiography, the main two questions to be asked are:

  i. Is the size of the ventricle and its walls normal?
 ii. What is the systolic function of the left ventricle?

If there is reduced systolic function, it is likely to be due to either abnormality in systolic contraction in a specific region or a global process where the entire left ventricle is impaired. The size of the left ventricle is conventionally measured in the parasternal long-axis view, between the interventricular septum and the anterolateral wall (normal values: women 3.8–5.2 cm and men 4.2–5.8 cm), at the level of the mitral valve tips, in end-diastole. It is also useful at this stage to measure the thickness of the septum and anterolateral walls to give an indication whether there is abnormal hypertrophy, as seen in conditions like hypertensive heart disease and hypertrophic cardiomyopathies (HCM). This should also be assessed in end-diastole. For wall thickness, normal values are 0.6–0.9 cm for women and 0.6–1.0 cm for men. End-diastole is usually determined by simultaneous echo- and electrocardiographic assessment. Thinning of the myocardium is seen in regions and most commonly reflects regions of transmural myocardial infarction. The left ventricle may be globally thinned and dilated in severe ischaemic as well as dilated cardiomyopathies and in valvular heart disease (see **Figure 5.13**).

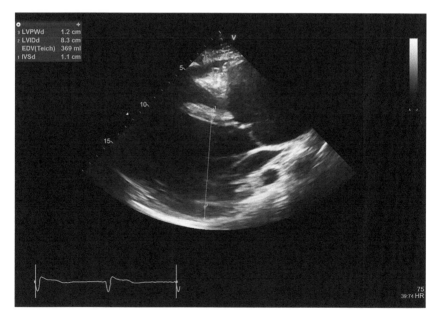

Figure 5.13 Image of dilated LV measuring 8.3 cm in diastole in a patient with a dilated aortic root and severe aortic regurgitation.

When judging whether overall ejection fraction is normal, wall motion should be compared in two perpendicular long-axis views. By convention the 2- and 4-chamber apical views used in echocardiography are used to measure ejection fraction. This can be assessed visually as the percentage of the end-diastolic volume (represented by area of ventricular cavity) which is ejected by the end of systole. As a rule of thumb, >50% is considered normal, 40%–50% mildly reduced, 30%–40% moderately reduced and <30% severely reduced. Ideally, ejection fraction is evaluated using Simpson's biplane method in systole and diastole across the apical 2- and 4-chamber views (see **Figure 5.14**).

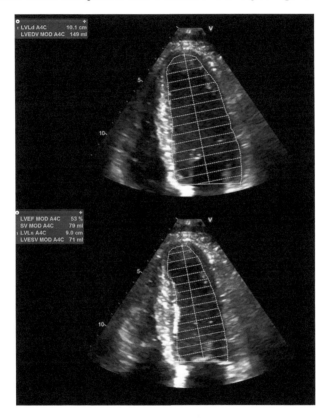

Figure 5.14 Illustration showing assessment of ejection fraction in the apical 4-chamber view in diastole (above) and systole (below).

If myocardial systolic dysfunction appears regional, as is seen in the context of myocardial infarction, it is important to identify the affected territory (see **Figure 5.15**).

A region of myocardium may be classified as normal, hypokinetic (reduced systolic movement), akinetic (absent movement), dyskinetic (paradoxical movement, i.e., outward movement during systole) or aneurysmal. When assessing for wall motion, it is useful to view the ventricle in the short-axis

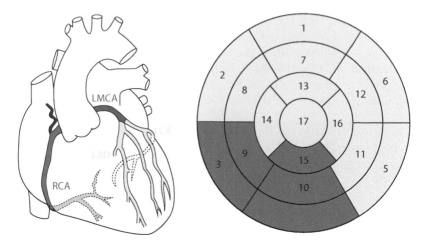

Figure 5.15 Seventeen-segment model showing which coronaries supply each region. (LMCA – left main coronary artery; LCX – left circumflex artery; LAD – left anterior descending artery; RCA – right coronary artery.)

views, comparing different segments against each other. The anteroseptum, anterior wall and apex are typically supplied by the left anterior descending (LAD) artery, the inferoseptum and inferior wall by the right coronary artery (RCA) and the inferolateral wall by the left circumflex (LCX) artery (although variations in coronary anatomy mean that this is not always the case).

Right Ventricle

Right ventricular morphology, size and function can be assessed in multiple views, but is perhaps best visualised in the 4-chamber apical view, as well as the 4-chamber subcostal view. This has the added benefit of being able to make direct comparison with the adjacent left ventricle. First, assess right ventricular size, which should be approximately two-thirds the size of the left ventricle and usually reflects a qualitative assessment. Right ventricular dilatation is always pathological. Formal dimensions are measured at the tricuspid valve annulus, mid-cavity in the parallel plane and longitudinally from the tricuspid annulus to the right ventricular apex. Normal right ventricular diameter is 1.9–3.5 cm at the mid-cavity level for both women and men (see **Figure 5.16**).

Measuring right ventricular function can be complex, but in the context of point-of-care echocardiography it is often done simply by a visual assessment of ejection fraction. Notice that the right ventricle exhibits both radial and longitudinal contraction, and that the latter is more marked in the right than the left ventricle. If right ventricular systolic function is reduced, it is sometimes possible to appreciate reduced movement of the tricuspid annulus

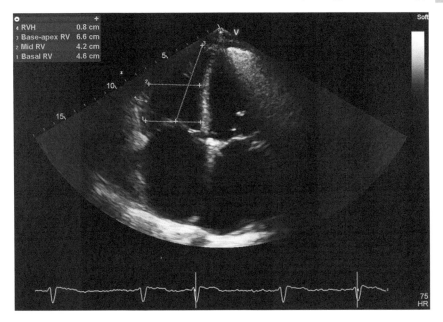

4 RVH	0.8 cm
3 Base-apex RV	6.6 cm
2 Mid RV	4.2 cm
1 Basal RV	4.6 cm

Figure 5.16 Patient with dilated right heart and corresponding measurements.

towards the apex during systole, although this takes experience to appreciate. As a rule of thumb, a right ventricular ejection fraction of >50% can be considered normal. In acute right ventricular decompensation due to massive pulmonary embolus, the right ventricle is often dilated.

Atria

Left atrial size is seen best in the apical 4-chamber view. It has relevance because it may be clearly dilated in atrial fibrillation, mitral valve disease, cardiomyopathy or a combination of these pathologies. A left atrial diameter of 2.7–3.8 mm in women and 3.0–4.0 mm in men can be considered normal. Assessment of the right atrium has a less prominent role in point-of-care echocardiography, but visual appreciation of its size and function is still possible, again predominantly from the apical 4-chamber view. Amongst the pathological processes causing dilatation of the right atrium are severe tricuspid regurgitation, atrial septal defects, atrial fibrillation and pulmonary hypertension (see **Figure 5.17**).

Valves

Aortic Valve

The aortic valve is situated at the junction of the left ventricular outflow tract and the aorta. As described previously, it can be characterised in parasternal

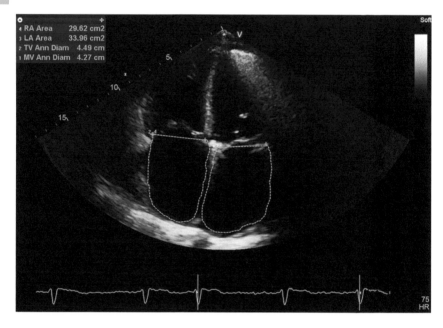

Figure 5.17 Apical 4-chamber view showing bi-atrial dilatation.

long- and short-axis orientations, as well as the apical 5-chamber view. In the context of point-of-care echocardiography, the main aims are to describe the anatomy of the valve and identify if there is valve dysfunction resulting from either aortic stenosis or aortic regurgitation contributing to the clinical presentation. The aortic valve has three cusps (also known as leaflets) behind which the aortic wall bulges into the sinus of Valsalva. The right coronary cusp is located anteriorly, so-called as the right coronary artery arises from the aortic wall behind the valve leaflet. The left and non-coronary cusps are located posteriorly, the aorta behind which giving rise to the left main stem and abutting the interatrial septum respectively. Valve opening can be visually assessed, whereby the valve orifice forms a uniform triangle shape in systole.

It is possible to see valvular calcification in this view, which can cause two of the leaflets to become fused and give rise to a stenotic lesion. Both stenotic and regurgitant lesions can further be characterised in the long-axis orientations. With the transducer in parasternal long-axis window, the ultrasound beam bisects the right coronary cusp anteriorly, then the non-coronary cusp and left atrium posteriorly. Notice the sinuses of Valsalva behind the valve leaflets. The valve leaflets should open widely in systole and close uniformly in diastole. By placing colour Doppler over the valve, turbulent forward flow in conjunction with restricted opening is indicative of aortic stenosis, where a regurgitant jet of backflowing blood will be seen in aortic regurgitation. If the regurgitation is severe and secondary to a rupture or flail leaflet, prolapse of one of the aortic valve leaflets may be evident (**Figure 5.18**).

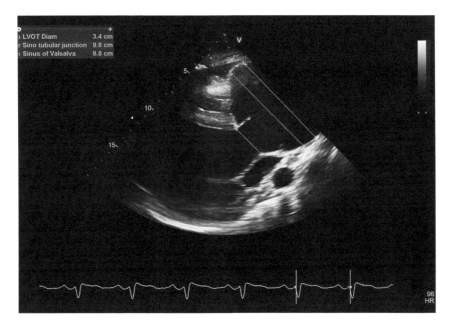

Figure 5.18 Dilated aortic root in a patient with severe aortic regurgitation. This image shows the aortic root at the sinus of Valsalva measuring at 10 cm.

Mitral Valve

The mitral valve, situated between the left atrium and left ventricle, is a complex anatomical structure consisting of the mitral annulus, two valve leaflets (anterior and posterior) and the sub-valvular apparatus (chordae tendineae and papillary muscle insertions). The valve is well-characterised in the parasternal long- and short-axis views. In the long-axis view, the image plane bisects the anterior and posterior leaflets, allowing visual appreciation of valve opening during diastole and rapid closure in systole.

Similar to aortic valve assessment, applying colour Doppler enables visual appreciation of regurgitant forward flow back into the left atrium in systole and, although it is more unusual, turbulent flow of mitral stenosis in diastole. A variety of pathology can cause mitral regurgitation including annular dilatation due to left ventricular failure (known as functional mitral regurgitation), endocarditis where vegetative lesions prevent effective valve closure and chord or papillary muscle rupture which can occur as a complication of

67

myocardial infarction. In papillary or chord rupture, the untethered mitral valve apparatus is seen freely moving within the left ventricular cavity and the affected leaflet may be seen to prolapse through the mitral annulus into the left atrium (flail leaflet), where regurgitation will often be severe. Next rotate the probe to assess the mitral valve in the short axis for visualisation of leaflet opening and closure. Restricted opening of mitral stenosis as well as morphological anomalies may be appreciable.

Right Heart Valves

Tricuspid valve assessment is central to estimation of pulmonary arterial pressures in conventional echocardiography. For point-of-care assessment, however, it is simply important to recognise severe regurgitation and major structural abnormalities affecting the valve. As well as the long-axis 4-chamber views, the parasternal long-axis view with tricuspid tilt enables visualisation of the tricuspid valve, and the principles described previously apply to its assessment. Colour Doppler can help to characterise significant regurgitation, which may be a primary cause (e.g., endocarditis, rheumatic, chord rupture, congenital) or secondary cause (e.g., pulmonary hypertension, pulmonary valve disease, right heart failure, ischaemic). Whilst the pulmonary valve may be seen in parasternal axis view with tricuspid tilt and parasternal short-axis view, formal assessment with point-of-care echocardiography is challenging. If it is well-visualised, colour Doppler may reveal significant stenosis or regurgitation, pointing to the need for more formal quantitative study.

Vegetations

Vegetations are lesions which form on a heart valve, consisting of fibrin, platelets, inflammatory cells and colonies of micro-organisms where they occur in the context of infective endocarditis (as is most common). They can occur on any of the heart valves and can cause both stenotic and regurgitant lesions which may be detectable before the vegetation becomes visible with imaging (often only when they reach 2 mm in size). Identification and diagnosis are important as some organisms are highly destructive of the valve apparatus, and imaging characteristics can be helpful to guide further investigation and management. Existing valvular lesions and any prosthesis are at increased risk of developing infective endocarditis. In the context of point-of-care echocardiography, the main aims of imaging are to identify macroscopic vegetation material on the valves, detect complications resulting from a vegetation and identifying indications for urgent surgery (severe valve regurgitation or obstruction, aortic root dilatation and cardiac failure resulting from the valve lesion). Vegetations may be fixed to the valve apparatus or attached by a pedicle and freely mobile throughout the cardiac cycle. Transthoracic echocardiography has lower sensitivity to detect vegetations and depending on the degree of clinical suspicion of endocarditis, most patients will undergo transoesophageal echocardiography.

Inside/Outside of the Heart

In addition to assessment of systolic and valvular function, point-of-care echocardiography can be used to look at structures within and around the heart, predominantly the pericardium, aorta and cardiac masses, as well as to assess venous pressure and fluid status.

Venous Pressure and Fluid Status

Using the subcostal window as described previously, the inferior vena cava can be seen within the liver and where it connects with the right atrium. With respiration its diameter varies, decreasing in calibre with inspiration in normal physiology, remaining persistently increased throughout respiration in right heart pressure and volume overloaded states, and paradoxically increasing with inspiration in restrictive physiology, the Kussmaul effect. As a general rule, an inferior vena cava diameter of 1.5–2.5 cm can be considered normal and collapses up to 50% with inspiration. Less than 1.5 cm diameter indicates underfilling, >2.5 cm with and without collapse indicates increasing degrees of overfilling with raised right-sided pressures.

Pericardium

The pericardial sac surrounds the heart and consists of an outer fibrous layer, with an inner serous layer of which a parietal layer adheres to the outer fibrous layer and an inner visceral layer adheres to the heart. Between the two layers of the serous pericardium there is a potential space, which normally contains a small rim of pericardial fluid. Pericardial disease can cause fluid to build up in this space which can affect the functioning of the heart. The normal fibrous pericardium is relatively bright on echocardiography, with any fluid within the pericardium appearing black. The pericardial space can be assessed in virtually all echocardiography windows, and it will depend on where any increase in pericardial fluid is located as to which view is optimal. The subcostal view is a good place to start.

Although a clinical diagnosis, recognising signs of tamponade is a key utility of point-of-care cardiac ultrasound. When an effusion reaches a size sufficient enough to cause compression and impair cardiac filling, the cardiac output will begin to be compromised. In addition to the clinical signs of tamponade, the presence of a pericardial effusion in conjunction with diastolic collapse of the right atrium and ventricle demonstrate the pressure effect of the fluid on cardiac filling, resulting in cardiac tamponade physiology. When the pressure effect is alleviated by drainage of the pericardial fluid, it is the right ventricular filling which normalises first, demonstrating impaired right atrial filling to be an earlier marker of impending tamponade.

Aorta

The aorta above the valve can be seen in the parasternal long-axis and apical 5-chamber view, and the arch and its branches may be visible using the suprasternal window. Point-of-care echocardiography aims to identify two aortic pathologies: aortic aneurysm and aortic dissection. Aneurysm of the ascending aorta can be seen and measured in the parasternal long-axis view. This may or may not be associated with abnormal aortic valve morphology and function (see **Figure 5.18**).

Aortic dissection, where the intima tears allowing blood to track down a false lumen, is most accurately characterised on transoesophageal echocardiography or computed tomography imaging. Dissection of the aortic root or arch (Type A) may be detected by transthoracic point-of-care echocardiography, however, it is important to state that absence of dissection cannot rule it out. When imaging the dissection of the aortic root or arch, a dissection flap may be visible at the site of the tear and a separate false lumen may be demonstrated.

Thrombus

Mural thrombus occurs relatively frequently as a complication of myocardial infarction, particularly following extensive anterior territory infarction, but can also occur in cardiomyopathy states where the left ventricular function is severely impaired. Where segments are akinetic, blood pools and thrombus form there, posing a risk of systemic embolic phenomena. Ventricular thrombus is most commonly seen at the apex and as such can be easily missed on transthoracic echocardiography. Thrombus is also common in the left atrium and left atrial appendage. Although it is not possible to adequately interrogate the appendage with transthoracic echocardiography, thrombus may arise from other structures within the atria, especially in the context of atrial fibrillation. Thrombus usually appears bright but can also appear with similar echodensity to myocardium. It can be adhered to the myocardial wall and appear immobile, but equally manifest as a large mobile thrombus arising from a defect in the interatrial septum. Colour Doppler may help to distinguish thrombus from stagnant blood flow.

Tumours

Due to the crossover in imaging characteristics, it is important to consider cardiac tumours in the differential for thrombus. Whilst rare, tumours of the heart can present in a variety of ways and echocardiography is an ideal first-line assessment to help guide further investigation, which often involves multiple imaging modalities. Whether primary or secondary (as is more common), malignant or benign, there is no 'one-size-fits-all' approach with echocardiography of cardiac tumours. Some may be very apparent, highly mobile in the blood pool and well-demarcated from other cardiac structures; others are poorly differentiated and difficult to distinguish from the myocardium. The aim of point-of-care echocardiography is not to provide a definitive diagnosis, but rather to detect features which may indicate a cardiac neoplastic process. Myxomas are the most common cardiac tumour, usually arising from the left side of the interatrial septum (although other origins are recognised). They are not malignant but can become significantly large to cause haemodynamic compromise, as well as provide a surface on which thrombus can form. They are frequently mobile and well-demonstrated in echocardiographic windows where the atria are well-characterised. Colour Doppler may identify larger blood vessels within a highly vascular lesion.

Conclusion

Point-of-care echocardiography offers a readily available, portable and highly versatile assessment of a wide variety of cardiac pathologies. Being patient, focussing on patient positioning, echocardiography windows and acoustic conduction are all key to achieving high quality and successful imaging. Using a systematic approach will also pay dividends and save time. With training and practise, point-of-care echocardiography can be an immensely valuable tool in the acute assessment of unstable patients to help guide their immediate management.

CHAPTER 6

ABDOMINO-PELVIC ULTRASOUND

Kirsten MS Kind

Learning Objectives

- Understand the abdominal and pelvic anatomy relevant for ultrasound assessment.
- Appreciate the importance of a systematic approach.
- Be able to assess individual organs and recognise key abnormalities.
- Be familiar with common pathologies.
- Recognise the limitations of ultrasound and when to consider other specialist investigations.

Anatomy

There are many different structures within the abdominal and pelvic cavities, and a solid grasp of the anatomy is vital to obtaining and interpreting diagnostic images of these regions (see **Figures 6.1** and **6.2**). The liver is the largest organ within the abdomen and lies in the right upper quadrant, abutting the right hemidiaphragm. It usually lies, at least partially, above the costal margin, making it harder to evaluate in its entirety. Tucked under the liver is the gallbladder, which drains via the cystic duct into the common bile duct (CBD). The common bile duct is formed when the intra-hepatic bile ducts and the cystic duct converge at the hepatic hilum and is an important structure to evaluate in ultrasound assessment of the acute abdomen. The spleen occupies the left upper quadrant, abutting the left hemidiaphragm, and is usually smaller than the liver. In the midline, the pancreas sits beneath the stomach, draped over the splenic vein, and comprises a head, body and tail. Inferior and deep to the pancreas in the midline pass the aorta and inferior vena

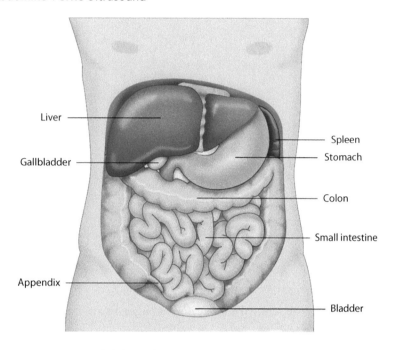

Figure 6.1 Overview of abdominal anatomy.

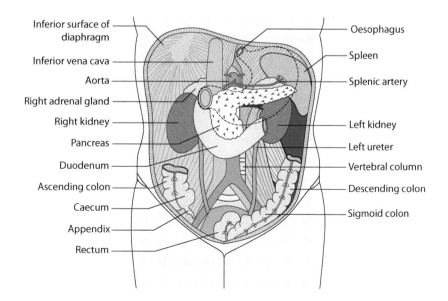

Figure 6.2 Retroperitoneal structures.

cava. The kidneys are situated laterally and posteriorly and are often easiest to visualise from the back or side of the patient. The right kidney sits slightly more inferiorly than the left, thanks to the bulky liver lying just above it. The ureters exit the kidneys at the renal hila and pass inferiorly to enter the urinary bladder supero-posteriorly. The bladder should lie centrally within the pelvis.

In female patients, the uterus is positioned between the bladder and the rectum in the sagittal plane and should be in the midline. The ovaries may vary in their position, but should always lie within the pelvic cavity, with one on either side of the uterus. The large bowel lies in the periphery of the abdomen, starting with the caecum in the right iliac fossa and progressing through the ascending, transverse, descending and sigmoid colon through to the rectum in the pelvis. The appendix arises from the caecum. The small bowel lies predominantly centrally in the abdomen, arising from the gastric outlet and comprises (proximal to distal) the duodenum, jejunum and ileum. The small bowel joins the large bowel at the ileocaecal valve in the right iliac fossa.

Systematic Approach to Assessment

A systematic approach is important in all areas of imaging, but especially when evaluating an area with so many different important structures. In this section I will outline the approach that I was taught, and still use to this day. However, should you find a different order works for you, then stick with that. The important thing is to make sure that you cover each of these areas in your system; the order doesn't really matter.

1. Liver
   a. Longitudinal sweep
   b. Transverse sweep
2. Gallbladder
3. Common bile duct (CBD)
4. Right kidney
5. Pancreas
6. Aorta
7. Spleen
8. Left kidney
9. Urinary bladder
10. Appendix*
11. Uterus*
12. Ovaries*

This system follows a logical progression from the right upper quadrant, across the midline to the left upper quadrant, then down to the pelvis.

---

* If appropriate.

Obviously, if you are only interested in a particular system (urinary tract, female reproductive organs, etc.) then you can target your examination appropriately. I would, however, recommend performing a full abdominal and pelvic examination whenever time allows, primarily to help you practice.

Specific Organ Assessment

Liver

Anatomy

The liver is the largest organ in the abdominal cavity and, thanks to its high position in the right hypochondrium/upper quadrant, it can be difficult to evaluate thoroughly on ultrasound. The liver is divided into segments (see **Figure 6.3**), which can be extremely useful when describing a focal abnormality. The caudate lobe (segment 1) is the portion of the liver parenchyma immediately adjacent to the inferior vena cava (IVC). The left lobe of the liver is divided into segments 2, 3 and 4. The larger right lobe is divided into segments 5 to 8. Each segment is delineated in the horizontal plane by the portal veins and in the vertical plane by the left, middle and right hepatic veins. The falciform ligament runs between segments 2/3 and 4. Getting your head around the segmental anatomy can be tricky, but well worth the time.

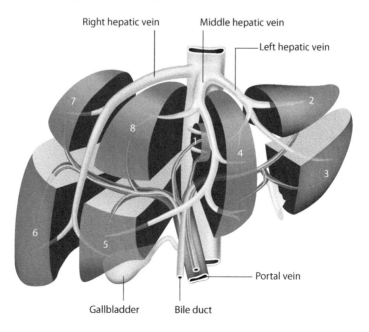

Figure 6.3 Segmental anatomy of the liver.

Technique

Start by using a curvilinear probe in a mid-frequency range but be ready to change to a lower frequency if your patient is very large. Place the probe in a craniocaudal (longitudinal) plane in the right upper quadrant, just below the costal margin. This should give you a sagittal image roughly in the middle of the liver (see **Figure 6.4**).

At this point, ask the patient to take a deep breath in (if they can) and hold it. This pushes the diaphragm down, bringing the liver below the costal margin, and makes it easier to see. While the patient holds their breath, sweep left and right with your probe (by tilting, rather than moving the probe) and take plenty of stills or a cine loop as you go. Make sure you see the left and right edges of the liver. Don't forget to tell the patient they can breathe away when you're done! Now turn your probe 90° to achieve an axial (transverse) view. Ask the patient to take another deep breath in and do another sweep, this time up and down, again taking plenty of still images or a cine loop as you go. Again, make sure you see the top and bottom edges of the liver. Tell the patient to breathe away. These two sweeps should hopefully give you a good view of the majority of the liver parenchyma. If anything catches your eye, you can focus in on the area by moving your probe but bear in mind that you may need to look through a window between ribs (angle your probe in line with the ribs). Now try to obtain an image with the liver parenchyma

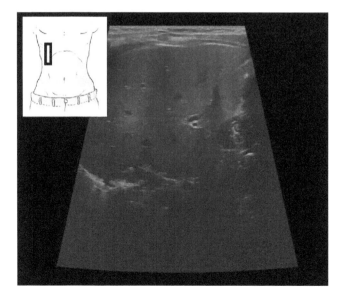

Figure 6.4 Liver visualised in sagittal section using ultrasound probe in longitudinal plane.

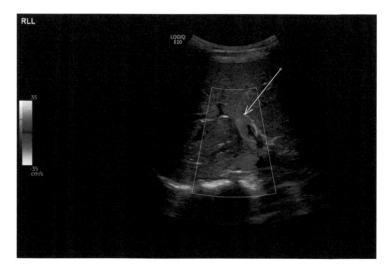

Figure 6.5 Colour Doppler flow in red showing the portal vein flowing *into* the liver.

adjacent to the right kidney – the two organs should be of similar echogenicity. If the kidney looks very dark compared to the liver, that can be a sign of fatty infiltration of the liver and is important to note.

Use the colour Doppler function to evaluate flow in the portal vein. This structure will be hypoechoic (dark) like other fluid-filled vessels and you'll see it entering the liver at the hepatic hilum. Centre your Doppler box over the hilum and look for a nice, constant flow *into* the liver (see **Figure 6.5**). The power Doppler function can be used to generate a waveform if you need further confirmation. Portal vein flow can be reversed in conditions such as liver cirrhosis, so it is important to assess this vessel routinely. Doppler can also be used to evaluate the hepatic veins (which flow *out* of the liver into the inferior vena cava) and the hepatic artery (which flows *into* the liver, alongside the portal vein), although these tend to form part of a more subspecialist workup, for example in liver transplant patients.

Gallbladder

Hopefully, during your sweeps of the liver, you will have identified the gallbladder. The gallbladder empties when we eat fatty foods, to release bile and help us break down that fatty food. For this reason, we ask all patients to fast for their ultrasound (usually for a minimum of 4 hours) to make sure the gallbladder is well-distended. Place your probe in the same place as you did for the liver, longitudinally in the right upper quadrant. If you can't see the gallbladder easily from here, tilting the patient slightly onto their left side can help. Try to get nice

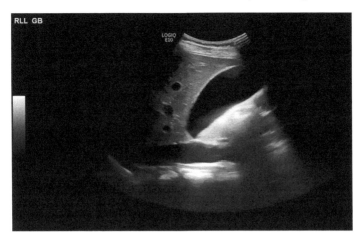

Figure 6.6 Normal gallbladder filled with hypoechoic bile.

longitudinal and transverse views of the gallbladder where you see the whole wall and the neck, as gallstones can get wedged there. A normal gallbladder is thin-walled (<3 mm), filled with uniformly hypoechoic material and should demonstrate posterior acoustic enhancement (see **Figure 6.6**).

Common Bile Duct (CBD)

The CBD exits the liver at the hepatic hilum, and you should be able to find it alongside the portal vein (see **Figure 6.7**). It can be tricky to tell apart from

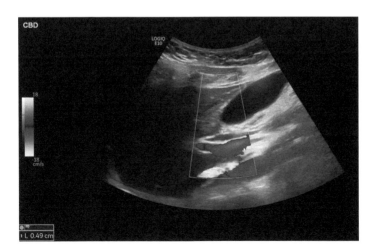

Figure 6.7 0.49 cm CBD visible at the hepatic hilum.

the adjacent vessels on grey-scale images, so put on your colour Doppler if you are not sure. Measure the CBD diameter and save this image. A rough guide for normal CBD calibre is:

CBD diameter (mm) = first digit of patient's age

For example, an 86-year-old man may have a normal CBD measuring 8 mm, while in a 40 year old the maximum would be 4 mm. Patients who have had their gallbladder removed (cholecystectomy) often have a dilated CBD as part of their normal postoperative anatomy, so don't apply this rule in those patients. If the CBD is wider than it should be, this usually implies an obstruction distally. Try to follow the CBD towards the ampulla as far as you can; you might spot a gallstone stuck in the duct. This is often tricky though, so don't worry if you don't see anything further down. These patients usually go onto specialist MRI imaging under the care of general surgeons.

Right Kidney

The right kidney is in the right flank, and you should have already seen it briefly during your evaluation of the liver. Place your probe in the right flank, just below the costal margin, and angle your probe to make the kidney as long as you can. Again, asking the patient to take a deep breath in can be helpful here. This gives you a longitudinal image of the kidney and allows you to measure the bipolar length if needed. Sweep through the kidney in this plane (by tilting your probe, not moving it) and make sure you see the whole organ. Then, rotate your probe by 90° to achieve a transverse view. Again, sweep through the kidney from top to bottom, taking plenty of saved images as you go. Be sure to stop at the midpoint to get a measurement of the renal pelvis in transverse (see **Figure 6.8**), as this allows you to assess objectively for hydronephrosis (dilation of the urine collecting system).

Pancreas/Aorta

These midline structures can be difficult to see on ultrasound, especially if the transverse colon is filled with gas. Start with your probe in the transverse plane, and position it centrally, just below the sternum (see **Figure 6.9**). Angle upwards slightly, towards the patient's head, and you should see the pancreas as a mid-echogenicity structure, lying across a large black vessel which will be the aorta (see **Figure 6.10**). The pancreas is usually of similar echogenicity to the adjacent liver. If it is much brighter than the liver, this can be a sign of pancreatitis. Move your probe inferiorly and adjust your depth to look just anterior to the spine. This should give you a clear view of the aorta (look for

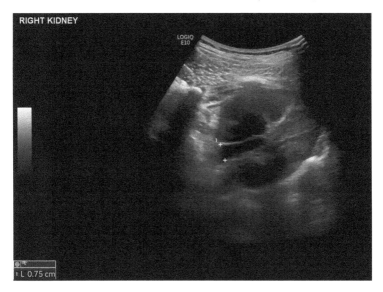

Figure 6.8 Transverse view of right kidney, with renal pelvis measured at 0.75 cm.

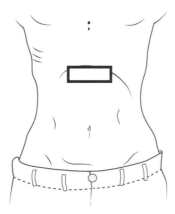

Figure 6.9 Position of ultrasound probe for assessing pancreas/aorta.

the pulsations to distinguish it from the neighbouring inferior vena cava). You should save both transverse and longitudinal images of the aorta and measure the diameter, looking out for abdominal aortic aneurysm. You may also identify other vascular structures in the vicinity of the pancreas including the superior mesenteric artery (SMA) and superior mesenteric vein (SMV) (see **Figure 6.11**).

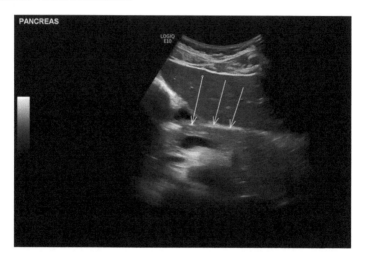

Figure 6.10 Ultrasound view of the pancreas (marked with thin white lines) lying beneath the liver and passing anterior to the left renal vein.

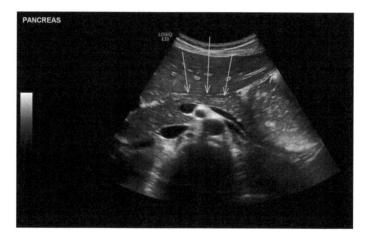

Figure 6.11 Second ultrasound view of pancreas with abdominal aorta, inferior vena cava (IVC), superior mesenteric artery (SMA), and superior mesenteric vein (SMV) all visible and seen to be lying underneath the left lobe of the liver and on top of the posteriorly placed vertebral body.

Spleen

To image the spleen, place your probe longitudinally in the left upper quadrant. You may have to ask the patient to breathe in to get a good view. Sweep through as you did for the liver and right kidney and try to get the whole organ on one image so that you can measure splenic size – splenomegaly (enlargement of the spleen) is an important finding to pick up (see **Figure 6.12**).

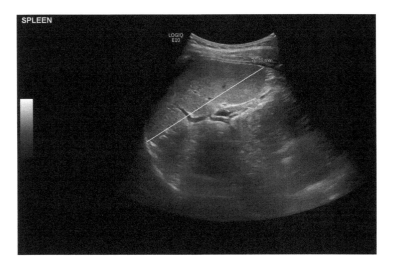

Figure 6.12 Ultrasound view of spleen measured at 78 mm.

Left Kidney

Approach the left kidney just as you did the right. Place the probe longitudinally in the left flank, angling to obtain the longest view of the kidney that you can. Sweep through from side to side, then rotate your probe by 90° and sweep from top to bottom. Don't forget to take plenty of images as you go along, including one of the renal pelvis in transverse to measure for hydronephrosis.

Urinary Bladder

The bladder lies centrally within the pelvis and is lower down than you may think. Making sure the patient's trouser/waistbands are lowered to the level of their pubic bone will make obtaining a good image much easier (see **Figure 6.13**). Asking your patient to have a full bladder is also essential to allow you to evaluate the bladder wall thoroughly. Place your probe in the transverse plane, low down in the central suprapubic region. You may have to reduce your gain here to reduce artefact in a full bladder. Be sure to get views of the bladder in both the transverse and longitudinal planes to allow measurement of pre- and post-micturition volumes if required (see **Figures 6.14–6.16**).

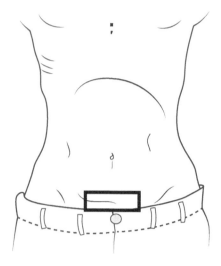

Figure 6.13 Position of ultrasound probe for visualising bladder/pelvic structures.

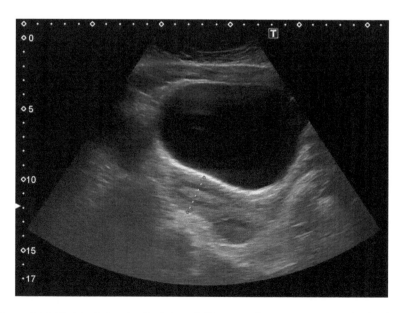

Figure 6.14 Bladder in longitudinal view. Callipers can be seen measuring the fundus of the uterus.

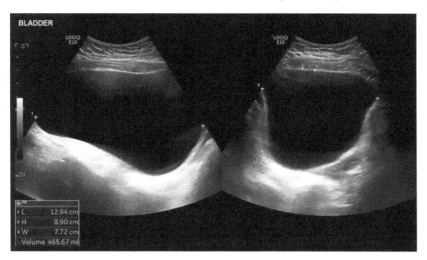

Figure 6.15 Bladder pre-micturition (bladder volume measured at 465 mls).

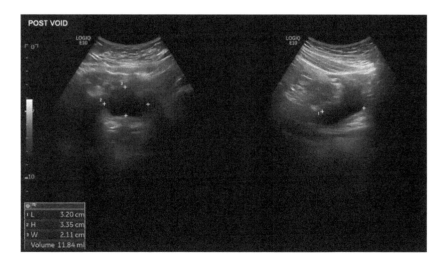

Figure 6.16 Bladder post-micturition (bladder volume measured at 11.8 mls).

Appendix

The appendix can be very difficult to identify on ultrasound, particularly in adult patients. The best way to spot it is to look for it on every abdominal or pelvic scan you perform to get used to the anatomy and to know what a normal appendix looks like. Place your probe in the transverse position in the

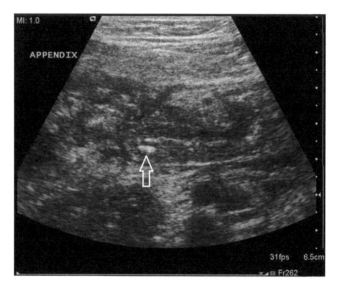

Figure 6.17 Appendix visualised in longitudinal section with appendicolith seen at tip (white arrow).

right flank and look for the ascending colon (often gas filled, so may reflect your ultrasound waves). Follow this inferiorly until you reach the caecum and look for a blind-ending tubular structure (see **Figure 6.17**). Once you have identified the appendix, you should measure its diameter and wall thickness, then look out for other features of appendicitis, such as hyperaemia (on Doppler), adjacent free fluid or an appendicolith (small focus of calcification in an infected appendix). If the total outer diameter is greater than 6 mm or the individual wall thickness is more than 3 mm, findings are in keeping with appendicitis (see **Figure 6.18**).

Female Pelvic Organs

The uterus and ovaries are particularly radiosensitive reproductive organs, which are not very well seen on CT, so they are often imaged using ultrasound in the first instance. Optimal images of these organs are obtained using a transvaginal probe, but this is a subspecialist area and beyond the scope of this book. Patient preparation is very important, and the patient should be asked to fill their bladder as much as possible prior to the examination. This allows a clear, fluid-filled 'window' through which to see the uterus and ovaries, as well as displacing the uterus posteriorly, making it easier to see. Effort should be made to obtain longitudinal and

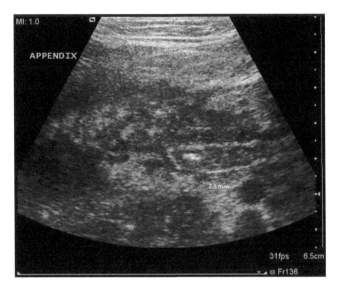

Figure 6.18 Same appendix measured at 7.8 mm in diameter in keeping with appendicitis.

transverse images of the uterus, similar to the kidneys, with a full sweep in each dimension. The ovaries can be difficult to see but should lie with one either side of the uterus in the transverse plane. Ovarian cysts are common and, if small and simple, may be physiological. If an ovarian cyst shows any concerning features (thick walls, internal septations, debris, large size), refer for specialist investigation.

Bowel

The bowel is, in general, difficult to assess with ultrasound, particularly in adult patients. If you are concerned about bowel pathology, ultrasound can be useful to look for secondary signs such as free fluid, but more definitive tests such as CT or MRI may be more appropriate.

Common Pathologies

The number of potential pathologies within the abdominal and pelvic cavities is vast and, as a rule, if you suspect something is not quite right during your bedside scan, referring the patient for further imaging in the radiology department is an essential next step. This final section includes still images from real patients and illustrates some of the more common pathologies that you are likely to come across in your practice.

Gallstones

Note the uniformly hypoechoic fluid within the gallbladder (bile) and the posterior acoustic shadowing (arrow) from the dense gallstones that are lying dependently (see **Figure 6.19**).

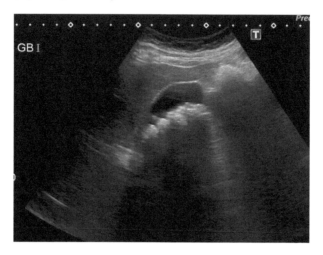

Figure 6.19 Gallstones contained within gallbladder.

Liver Haemangioma

Haemangiomata are well-circumscribed, hyperechoic lesions within the liver, often with increased vascularity on Doppler (see **Figure 6.20**).

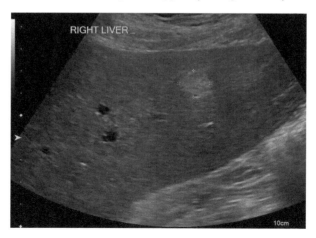

Figure 6.20 Haemangioma visualised within left lobe of liver.

Hydronephrosis

In the image in **Figure 6.21** we can see dilation of the proximal ureter (black arrow) as well as of the renal pelvis with blunting of the calyces (double white arrow).

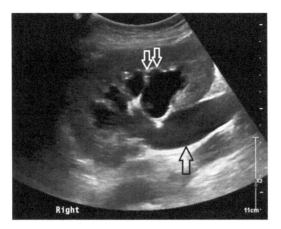

Figure 6.21 Hydronephrotic right kidney.

Ascites

The image in **Figure 6.22** is taken in the left iliac fossa, with several loops of collapsed/fluid-filled bowel (arrow) outlined by hypoechoic fluid, which shouldn't be there.

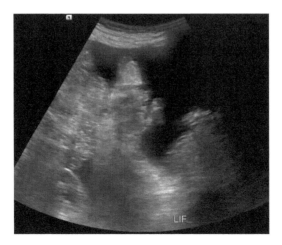

Figure 6.22 Ascitic fluid visible in left iliac fossa.

CHAPTER 7

MUSCULOSKELETAL ULTRASOUND

Kirsten MS Kind

Learning Objectives

- Understand the anatomy of the large joints (shoulder, hip, knee and ankle).
- Appreciate the fundamentals of carrying out an ultrasound assessment of the large joints.
- Be able to recognise the basic ultrasound appearance of the large joints.
- Be familiar with the ultrasound appearance of common joint pathology.

Introduction

The use of ultrasound in imaging the musculoskeletal (MSK) system is widespread and has a number of different applications. As most muscles, tendons and ligaments are superficial, they lend themselves to evaluation with high-frequency ultrasound, allowing dynamic interrogation of individual and groups of muscles during passive and active movement. It is also possible in certain situations to image joints for the presence of effusion and evidence of infection. Ultrasound can be a useful tool for guiding interventional procedures, such as biopsy or joint injection, and can even be used to evaluate the cortex of a bone to look for subtle fractures.

The scope of MSK ultrasound is so vast and, at times, technically challenging that it could not possibly be covered in its entirety in this chapter. The author hopes, therefore, to introduce you to the basic anatomy and principles used in imaging the large joints as may be relevant to point-of-care ultrasound for non-subspecialist practitioners.

The Hip Joint

Anatomy

The hip joint is a ball-and-socket joint, where the round head of the femur articulates with the acetabulum of the pelvis. A joint capsule encases the joint, which is lined by cartilage and synovium and contains a small volume of lubricating fluid. Several large muscles surround and support the hip joint, allowing multi-directional movement and enabling us to walk, run and jump. In two-legged mammals, the hips are the largest joints in the body, taking the weight of our upper body and distributing it evenly across our legs and feet. The most important anatomical landmark in ultrasound of the hip is the anterior recess – a 'pocket' between two layers of synovium at the anterior aspect of the femoral neck (see **Figure 7.1**).

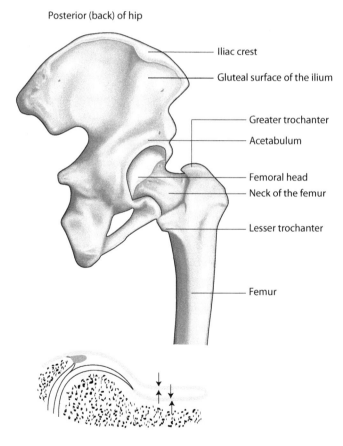

Posterior (back) of hip

Iliac crest

Gluteal surface of the ilium

Greater trochanter

Acetabulum

Femoral head

Neck of the femur

Lesser trochanter

Femur

Figure 7.1 The anatomy of the hip joint showing detail of joint capsule.

In the presence of a joint effusion, fluid is often seen within this recess, and ultrasound has been shown to be effective in detecting effusions in this manner. The primary role of ultrasound at the hip joint is to assess for the presence of a joint effusion and to guide aspiration of any excess fluid for cytology. In children, ultrasound is also used to assess the cartilaginous hips of the newborn for developmental dysplasia.

Technique

A linear transducer with a high-frequency range is ideal for smaller patients and children, but you may need to use lower-frequency curvilinear probes in larger adult patients. It is best to start with the highest-frequency probe and work your way down until you get good visualisation of the joint space and anterior recess in the middle of your field of vision. Orientation is vital to performing and interpreting ultrasound of the hip joint, so start off by positioning your probe on the patient in a sagittal plane. This should give you a longitudinal view of the femoral neck, allowing a clear view of the anterior recess (see **Figure 7.2**).

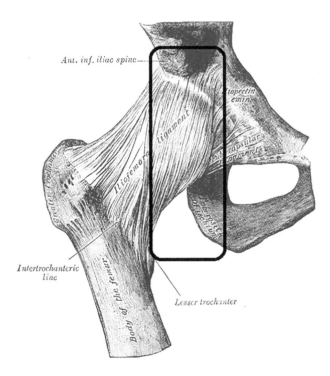

Figure 7.2 Demonstrating the correct probe positioning for imaging of the right hip joint.

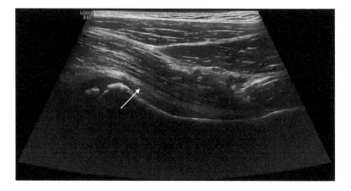

Figure 7.3 Normal hip joint. The anterior recess (arrow) is only just visible in the absence of excess joint fluid.

In a normal hip joint, the anterior recess will be barely visible, if at all (see **Figure 7.3**). However, in the presence of joint fluid, the anterior synovial lining will be lifted and a hypoechoic area will be visible between the overlying muscle and the bone surface (see 'Pathologies' section at the end of this chapter). It is also worth noting if the synovium appears thickened, and if there is debris within the effusion or simple, uniform hypoechoic fluid.

The Knee Joint

Anatomy

The knee joint is a synovial joint (lined with synovium and with a joint capsule) with one primary direction of movement (flexion/extension). The femur articulates with the tibia inferiorly and the patella anteriorly. The fibula articulates only with the tibia and is an important attachment site for some of the many stabilising ligaments of the knee. The patella is the largest sesamoid bone in the body, embedded within the quadriceps and patellar tendons which traverse the anterior aspect of the knee joint. Where the femoral condyles articulate with the tibial plateau are two menisci (medial and lateral), providing cushioning for this load-bearing joint and allowing a more even distribution of weight (see **Figure 7.4** for the relevant knee anatomy).

Several important ligaments stabilise the knee joint and are commonly injured, particularly in sportsmen and women. The cruciate ligaments cross centrally between the distal femur and proximal tibia in the intercondylar notch and provide anteroposterior stability. The medial and lateral collateral

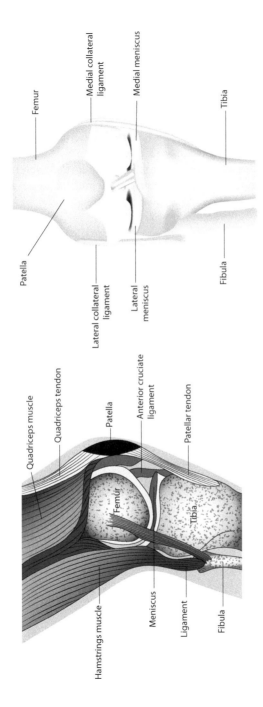

Figure 7.4 The anatomy of the knee joint.

ligaments run along the medial and lateral aspects of the joint, giving side-to-side stability. Though these structures are vital in investigating knee injury, they cannot be assessed by ultrasound and usually require MRI for full evaluation. The role of ultrasound is primarily in assessing the superficial anterior ligaments (quadriceps and patellar) and looking for joint effusion.

Technique

The approach to ultrasound of the knee joint is similar to that of the hip joint, and getting yourself orientated is key. Begin by placing your probe (a high-frequency linear array with a large footprint is preferable) longitudinally over the superior aspect of the knee joint in the midline (see **Figure 7.5**). This should give you a nice view of the quadriceps tendon, the superior aspect of the patella and the suprapatellar space (see **Figure 7.6**), a common site for effusion. If you do see an effusion in the suprapatellar space, rotate your probe 90° and take some images in the transverse plane with and without colour Doppler. If there is hyperaemia and synovial thickening, you should

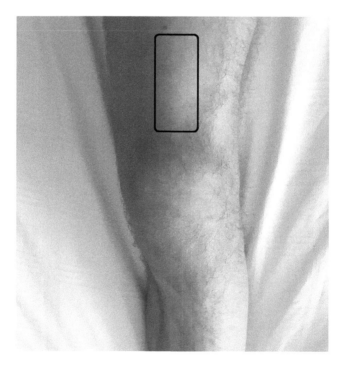

Figure 7.5 Probe positioning to begin ultrasound examination of the knee.

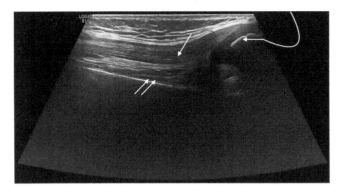

Figure 7.6 Superior knee joint, midline. Quadriceps tendon (arrow), suprapatellar space (double arrow) with no effusion and patella (curved arrow).

raise concerns of infected joint effusion/septic arthritis (see 'Pathologies' section at the end of this chapter).

If there is particular concern of Osgood-Schlatter disease (inflammation at the tibial tuberosity where the patellar tendon inserts), move your probe down to the tibial side of the joint, staying in the midline and in the longitudinal plane. Look for fluid around the patellar tendon insertion and put on colour Doppler to look for hyperaemia.

The Ankle Joint

Anatomy

The ankle joint refers to the articulation of the distal tibia and fibula with the dome of the talus (see **Figure 7.7**). The joint between the talus and the calcaneus is referred to as the subtalar joint. Numerous tendons and ligaments traverse and support the ankle and subtalar joint. In broad terms, the extensor tendons (responsible for extending or raising the toes) run across the superior aspect of the foot and anterior aspect of the ankle joint. The flexor tendons (responsible for flexing or curling the toes) pass along the sole of the foot and pass up the medial aspect of the ankle joint. Finally, the peroneal tendons (responsible for plantarflexing and everting the foot) pass across the sole of the foot and up the lateral aspect of the ankle joint. There are a number of other small ligaments between each of the bones of the hind- and midfoot, but those mentioned previously are the most relevant to your ultrasound examination. Like the hip and knee joints, the ankle joint is lined with synovium, so it can collect fluid in the form of an effusion.

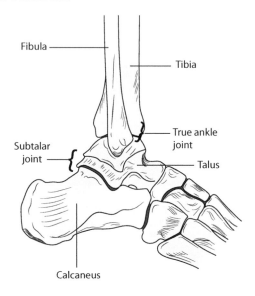

Figure 7.7 Basic anatomy of the ankle joint.

Technique

Complete structural and functional evaluation of the ankle joint is best undertaken by subspecialist sonographers and radiologists. It is possible, however, to look for an ankle joint effusion. Position the patient on the bed with their foot plantarflexed (toes pointed down) and place a linear, high-frequency probe over the anterior aspect of the ankle joint in the longitudinal plane (see **Figure 7.8**). This should afford you a view of the anterior aspect of the ankle joint and you should be able to see the distal tibia articulating with the dome of the talus (see **Figure 7.9**). An excess of hypoechoic fluid within the joint space is in keeping with an ankle joint effusion. Again, using colour Doppler to look for hyperaemia can be helpful to raise suspicion of septic arthritis.

Patients may present with focal areas of pain, redness or swelling on and around their ankle, and ultrasound is a really useful tool to evaluate specific areas of discomfort or abnormality. Place your high-frequency linear probe directly over the area of concern and be sure to use Doppler when interrogating the area. You may find thickening and hyperaemia of the superficial subcutaneous tissues, relating to cellulitis, or you may even find a foreign body. Your point-of-care ultrasound can be a great screening tool to guide further imaging, so if you see something that doesn't look right, send your patient for a dedicated departmental ultrasound for further investigation.

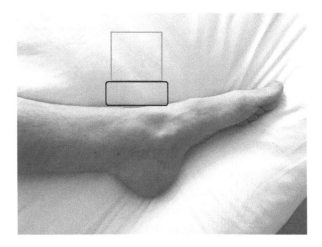

Figure 7.8 Positioning of probe to start ultrasound examination of ankle joint.

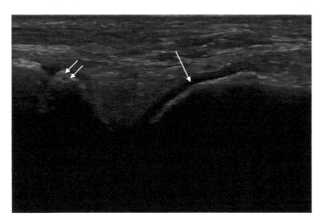

Figure 7.9 Anterior ankle joint. Distal tibia (double arrow) [with growth plate in this 12 year old] and dome of talus (arrow).

The Shoulder Joint

Anatomy

The shoulder is a ball-and-socket joint, with a supportive girdle of tendons and muscles allowing multi-directional movement (see **Figure 7.10**). Arguably the most important group of muscles at the shoulder are those of the rotator cuff. These muscles and tendons cross from the scapula to the bones of the forearm to support and facilitate movement at the shoulder. The supra- and infraspinatus muscles arise from the posterior surface of the scapula, extending across the

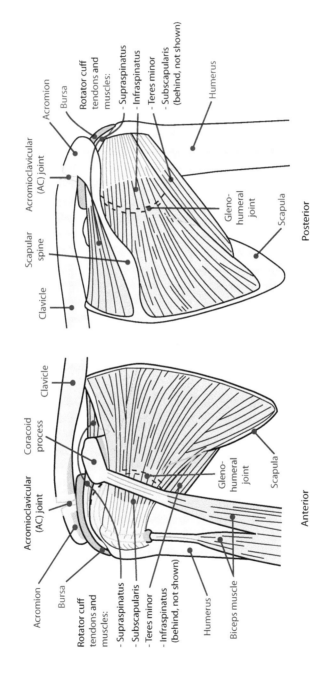

Figure 7.10 Anatomy of the shoulder joint.

glenohumeral joint to the humeral head. Teres minor is a smaller muscle, which passes inferior to the infraspinatus muscle from the lower border of the scapula to the humeral head. Finally, subscapularis arises from the anterior surface of the scapula and passes beneath the coracoid process to attach on the anterior surface of the humeral head. Together, these muscles and tendons make up the rotator cuff. Another important muscle of the arm is the biceps, whose tendons are an important part of shoulder movement. The tendon of the long head of the biceps attaches to the coracoid process, while the short head of the biceps tendon attaches to the anterior humeral head. Overlying all of these is a large superficial muscle, the deltoid. This muscle gives the shoulder its rounded shape, but is less often involved in pathology of the shoulder joint.

An experienced practitioner can usually tell from a detailed clinical examination which of these muscles or tendons are injured, allowing a focussed and systematic ultrasound to confirm the diagnosis. Of important note: ultrasound evaluation of the shoulder joint is a highly specialised examination and should only be performed by trained sonographers and radiologists. Unlike the other joints covered in this chapter, shoulder joint effusion is difficult to see on ultrasound and requires cross-sectional imaging or fluoroscopy to identify.

Pathologies (Figures 7.11–7.14)

Fluid in Biceps Tendon Sheath

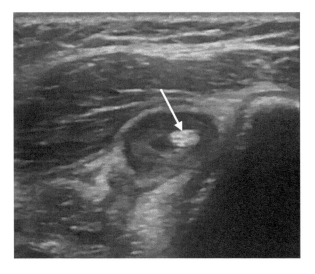

Figure 7.11 The hyperechoic biceps tendon (arrow) is seen here in cross-section and is surrounded by fluid and debris, indicating a shoulder joint septic arthritis.

Hip Effusion

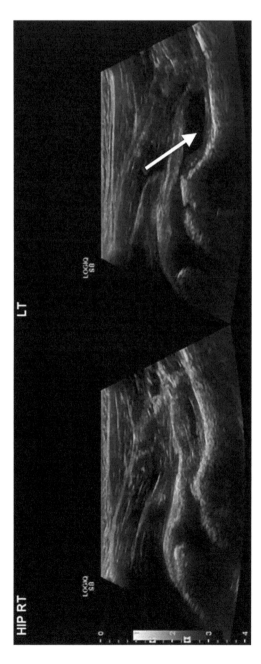

Figure 7.12 Comparison images of the right and left hip joints in a child. Note the fluid in the anterior recess on the left (arrow), raising the anterior synovium.

Knee Joint Effusion (Infected)

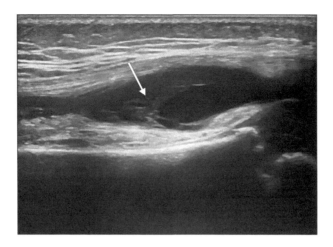

Figure 7.13 Longitudinal view of the suprapatellar space, which contains a complex, loculated fluid collection (arrow) indicative of septic arthritis.

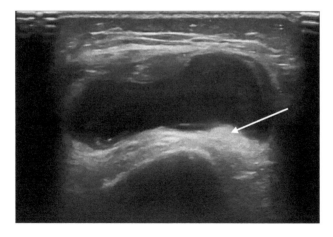

Figure 7.14 Same patient in transverse. Note the synovial thickening supporting the diagnosis of infected joint effusion/septic arthritis.

CHAPTER 8

ARTERIAL ULTRASOUND

James M Forsyth

Learning Objectives

- Appreciate the relevant arterial anatomy and common abbreviations for arteries used in vascular surgery and interventional radiology settings.
- Have a basic understanding of the common pathologies affecting the lower limb arterial system.
- Have a basic understanding of vascular duplex scanning modalities including grey-scale, colour Doppler and pulse wave Doppler.
- Be able to perform a basic lower limb arterial duplex assessment.

In this chapter, I will briefly cover a vascular surgery point-of-care ultrasound assessment of the lower limb arterial system. Importantly, this chapter represents an introductory foundation step into the world of arterial duplex scanning. The aim is to keep things simple, and we only venture slightly into the sophisticated world of ultrasound physics and specialist jargon. The purpose of this chapter is to keep things as simple as possible, captivate your interest and point you in the right direction. Note that in this chapter, I have focussed on using wireless ultrasound technology but the same principles apply when using standard ultrasound technology.

Arterial System

Anatomy

The main blood vessel arising from the heart is the thoracic aorta. After the aortic arch (which gives off the upper limb and carotid vessels), it descends through the chest as the descending thoracic aorta, and once it passes through the diaphragm it becomes the abdominal aorta. The abdominal aorta then splits to become the common iliac arteries, which split further to become the external and internal iliac arteries. The internal iliac arteries supply the pelvis/buttocks, and the external iliac arteries continue downwards to the groin beneath the inguinal ligament to become the common femoral arteries. The common femoral artery lies over the femoral head at the level of the groin, and just below here it splits into the superficial femoral artery and the profunda femoris artery or deep femoral artery. The profunda femoris artery mainly supplies the thigh, whilst the superficial femoral artery runs downwards toward the knee to supply the calf muscles. The superficial femoral artery becomes the popliteal artery as it passes through the adductor hiatus, then passes behind the knee. Above the knee, the popliteal artery is referred to as the *above-knee popliteal artery*, and below the knee it is referred to as the *below-knee popliteal artery*. The below-knee popliteal artery splits into three crural vessels: the posterior tibial artery, anterior tibial artery and peroneal artery. The anterior tibial artery passes from behind the knee through the interosseus membrane to run along the anterior shin and becomes the dorsalis pedis artery that lies in the forefoot lateral to the extensor hallucis longus tendon. See **Figure 8.1** for the relevant arterial anatomy.

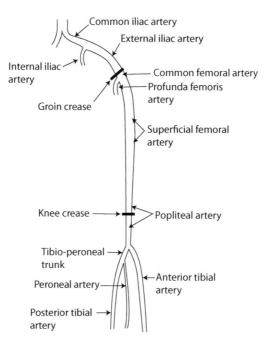

Figure 8.1 Basic lower limb arterial anatomy.

Here are some common abbreviations for the above arteries:

- External iliac artery – EIA
- Internal iliac artery – IIA
- Common femoral artery – CFA
- Superficial femoral artery – SFA
- Profunda femoris artery – PFA
- Above-knee popliteal – AK popliteal
- Below-knee popliteal – BK popliteal
- Anterior tibial artery – ATA
- Posterior tibial artery – PTA
- Tibioperoneal trunk – TPT (origin of the peroneal and posterior tibial arteries)

Basic Lower Limb Arterial Ultrasound Assessment

Preparation

- Introduce yourself to the patient and gain verbal consent to proceed.
- Wash your hands and clean the ultrasound probe with an alcohol wipe.
- Have a chaperone present throughout your assessment.
- Ask the patient to take his/her trousers, shoes and socks off and expose his/her abdomen.
- Position the patient in the supine position and ensure he/she is comfortable (provide a pillow for the patient's head to rest on and make sure the room temperature is satisfactory).
- The patient's leg/s should be slightly bent at the knee, with the hip slightly externally rotated and abducted.

Image Acquisition

- First, use the wireless ultrasound probe in grey-scale function to scan the mid-upper abdomen and screen for an abdominal aortic aneurysm (AAA). In a slim patient the high-frequency probe may be suitable. For larger patients the intermediate/lower-frequency probes will be needed to help you visualise the aorta at greater depth. If an aneurysm is present, clarify its size in the anterior-posterior (AP) dimension (see **Figure 8.2**). Adjust the depth, gain and focus on the ultrasound display to allow you to confidently visualise the abdominal aorta (the abdominal aorta is the deep structure lying at the back of the abdomen and resting directly on the vertebral bodies, so you will likely need to increase the

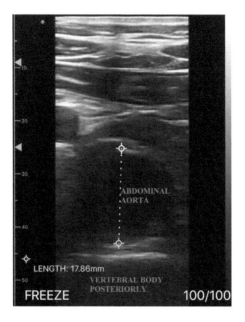

Figure 8.2 Normal-sized abdominal aorta in a thin patient (around 1.8 cm width). Note the posteriorly placed vertebral column.

depth, and position the focus much lower down). You may need to press downwards with the ultrasound probe to enable you to visualise the deeply positioned aorta.

- Move down to the groin and use the intermediate/higher-frequency ultrasound probe in either transverse or longitudinal orientation. Expect to have to re-adjust the depth and focus to make it more superficial. Use the grey-scale function to assess the CFA, along with the origins of the SFA and PFA (see **Figures 8.3–8.7**). Look for any gross evidence of disease, e.g., presence/absence of pulsation, strength of pulsation, calcification, plaque, thrombus, etc.

- Consider using colour Doppler to further clarify the CFA/SFA/PFA origins (see **Figures 8.8** and **8.9**). When using colour Doppler, you should steer the colour box to optimise your image (deliberately avoid a 90° angle of insonation). You can also adjust the pulse repetition frequency (PRF) button to optimise your image – this is to prevent something called *aliasing*. Aliasing is an imaging error which occurs when the sampling frequency is set too low, which therefore leads to assigning the incorrect colour to represent the velocity within the vessel. Also adjust the colour gain so that the colour flow is not spilling outward from the vessel walls (i.e., aim to keep the colour flow within the vessels).

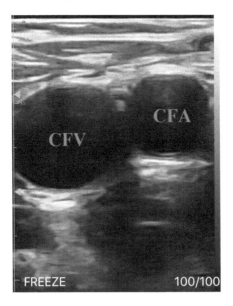

Figure 8.3 Normal CFA and adjacent common femoral vein (CFV) in transverse section. The artery has a thicker wall, is slightly smaller in size and has a more rounded appearance.

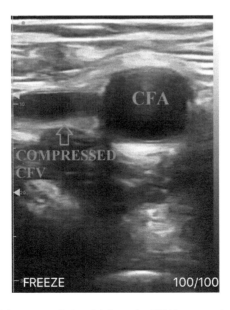

Figure 8.4 The CFA is easy to distinguish from the CFV because the vein compresses against the femoral head with little effort, whereas the artery does not.

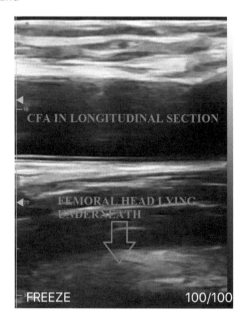

Figure 8.5 Normal CFA in longitudinal section lying directly over the femoral head.

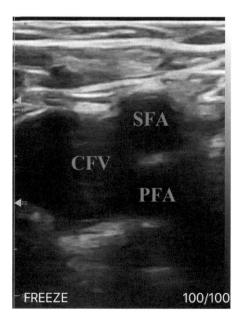

Figure 8.6 Normal SFA and PFA in transverse section just after they arise from the CFA.

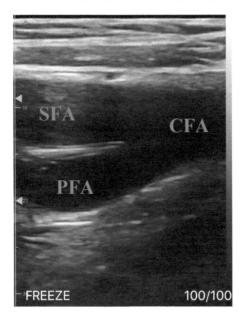

Figure 8.7 Normal SFA and PFA just after they arise from the CFA (longitudinal section).

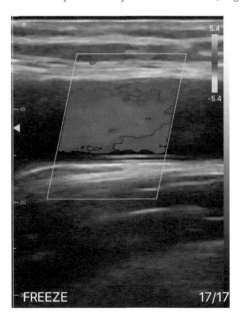

Figure 8.8 Normal CFA visualised in longitudinal section using colour Doppler. Note the colour box is slightly angled (by using the steer button).

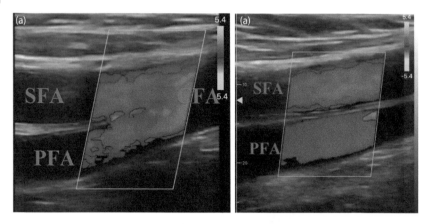

Figure 8.9 (a) Normal SFA and PFA arising from CFA in longitudinal section in colour Doppler; (b) the same SFA and PFA a few centimetres distal to their origins (further down the leg).

- Consider using pulse wave Doppler to assess the CFA/SFA/PFA origin waveforms. Distinguish between the three main types of arterial waveforms. Monophonic suggests severe arterial disease, biphasic suggests moderate arterial disease and triphasic suggests normal arterial flow (see **Figures 8.10** and **8.11**). A macroscopically normal appearing

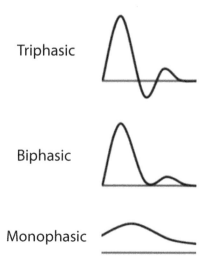

Figure 8.10 Image showing three different types of arterial waveforms that are identified using spectral Doppler.

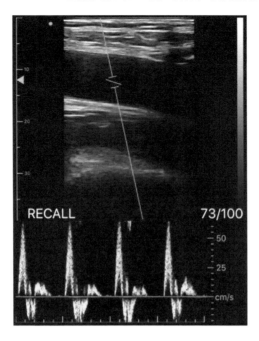

Figure 8.11 CFA origin in longitudinal section assessed using pulse wave Doppler (confirming normal triphasic flow). The angle and steer have been adjusted appropriately, with adjustment of wireless probe in head-toe position to align the CFA with the horizontal line.

artery with damped waveforms suggests more proximal disease (e.g., a normal appearing CFA with monophasic flow would suggest severe proximal iliac artery disease). When using pulse wave Doppler make sure to set the angle to $\leq 60°$, and avoid having the transducer steer at 90° because the Doppler shifts will not be coded. Adjust your head-toe wireless probe tilt so that the artery (in longitudinal section) aligns with the horizontal line (representing your angle). Also, adjust the pulse repetition frequency (PRF) button to optimise the waveform image. Finally, when assessing arteries, we recommend keeping the sample volume marker in the centre of the vessel and reducing the size of the sample volume to record mainly the maximum velocities in the centre of the vessel lumen.

▪ Now use the probe in longitudinal section to follow the SFA down toward the lower thigh. Assess individual sections, using a combination of grey-scale, colour Doppler and pulse wave Doppler. Keep the SFA visualised on the screen at all times and assess successive sections (see **Figures 8.12** and **8.13**).

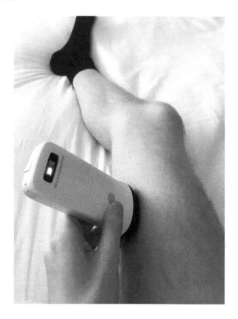

Figure 8.12 Position for scanning distal SFA/AK popliteal artery in longitudinal section.

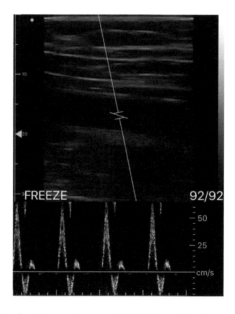

Figure 8.13 Triphasic flow in grossly normal SFA/AK popliteal artery.

- As already described, at the lower thigh level the SFA becomes the AK popliteal artery and dives into the adductor hiatus to follow a path behind the knee. Therefore, once you reach the lower part of the femur, move your ultrasound probe behind the knee and scan the artery here (see **Figure 8.14**). You will identify the BK popliteal artery. Again, check for size, pulsation and obvious disease in grey-scale function. Consider using colour Doppler and pulse wave Doppler to assess arterial flow (see **Figure 8.15**). To assess the popliteal artery with greater ease you can also ask the patient to roll over into the prone position.

- Beyond the BK popliteal artery, scanning the much smaller crural arteries is more advanced. For this basic introductory guide, we will just focus on two main areas: (1) the ATA at the ankle, and (2) the PTA at the ankle. By scanning these two areas you should be able to identify if there is significant crural vessel disease or not (see **Figures 8.16–8.20**). It is recommended to visualise these structures in longitudinal orientation and view the arteries in grey scale, then in colour Doppler and then finally using pulse wave Doppler.

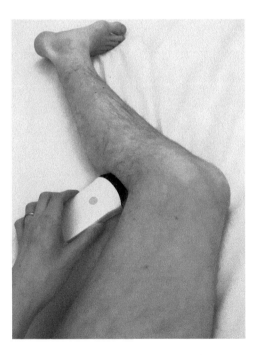

Figure 8.14 Wireless ultrasound probe held in longitudinal orientation behind the knee to assess the BK popliteal.

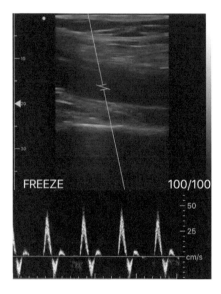

Figure 8.15 BK popliteal artery in longitudinal section demonstrating triphasic flow (note in this case the operator compressed the overlying popliteal vein in order to reduce the depth of the artery to improve the waveform signal).

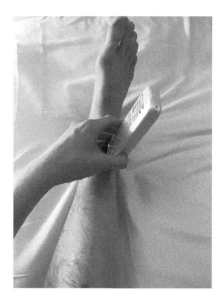

Figure 8.16 Wireless ultrasound probe in longitudinal section scanning AT artery at ankle level.

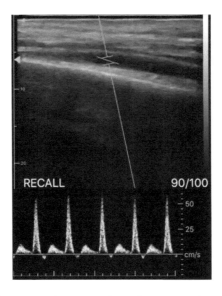

Figure 8.17 Normal AT artery showing triphasic flow using pulse wave Doppler.

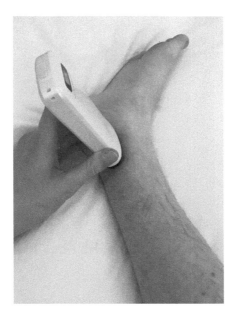

Figure 8.18 Wireless ultrasound probe in longitudinal section scanning PT artery at ankle level.

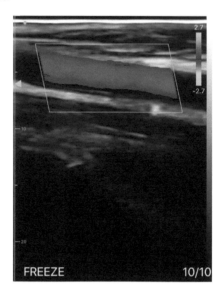

Figure 8.19 Normal PT artery using colour Doppler.

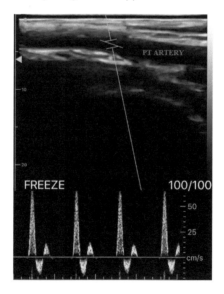

Figure 8.20 Normal PT showing triphasic flow using pulse wave Doppler.

Closing Steps

- Once you have completed your assessment, thank the patient and help remove the ultrasound gel from his/her skin.

- Wash your hands and cleanse the ultrasound probe with an alcohol wipe.
- Document your findings.
- Discuss your clinical and ultrasound findings with the patient.
- Decide upon further investigations/treatments as necessary.

Common Pathology Affecting Arterial System

The most common clinical indications for assessing the lower limbs in a vascular surgery context are:

1. Intermittent claudication
2. Chronic limb-threatening ischaemia
3. Acute limb ischaemia

Intermittent Claudication

When there is chronic stenotic or occlusive lower limb peripheral arterial disease, at the mild to moderate stage of the disease process, patients will present with symptoms on exercise. This is because at rest there is still sufficient blood supply to allow comfortable tissue perfusion. However, when the muscles are being exerted, the extra demand outweighs the deficient supply, and thus the patient experiences a cramping pain in the relevant muscle group. The symptoms are further exacerbated by going up an incline or stairs. Once the patient rests, the symptoms settle within a few minutes. This is called *intermittent claudication*. The muscle group that cramps is related to the site of the arterial disease. For example, with iliac artery disease the classical area for claudication pain is the buttock/thigh. For SFA disease the classical area for claudication pain is the calf. These patients may demonstrate signs of chronic low-level ischaemia, e.g., poor hair growth, muscle wasting.

Chronic Limb-Threatening Ischaemia

Chronic limb-threatening ischaemia (CLTI) represents the severe end of the arterial disease spectrum. The definition of CLTI is *ischaemic rest pain or tissue loss (ulceration or gangrene) for 2 weeks or more in the presence of atherosclerotic peripheral arterial disease.* These patients normally present with rest pain in the forefoot and with severe night pain in the forefoot that prevents them from sleeping. They often report having to sleep with the leg hanging out of bed (such that gravity can be used to help improve the foot blood supply and relieve their ischaemic pain). The diagnosis should also be associated with one or more abnormal hemodynamic parameters, e.g., a reduced ankle-brachial pressure index (ABPI) (<0.4).

Acute Limb Ischaemia

Acute limb ischaemia represents the sudden occlusion of a major lower limb artery and classically leads to the following signs and symptoms (6 Ps):

- Pain
- Pallor
- Pulselessness
- 'Perishingly' cold
- Paraesthesia
- Paralysis

The classic cause is a cardiac embolus in a patient with atrial fibrillation. The embolus is sent from the heart down the patient's aorta and lodges in a major lower limb vessel. Typical sites include the SFA, popliteal artery and/or the crural vessels. Sometimes a large embolus can lodge at the aortic bifurcation and lead to complete occlusion of both iliac arteries, resulting in bilateral lower limb ischaemia. Other embolic causes include a dislodged left ventricular thrombus following a large myocardial infarction or a proximal diseased artery that throws off thrombotic material. Other causes for consideration include a thrombosed popliteal aneurysm which can cause occlusion of the distal crural vessels, along with in situ thrombosis of a chronically diseased artery. It is also increasingly common to see patients who have previously had arterial bypass surgery or arterial stents to present with acutely ischaemic limbs when their bypasses/stents occlude. These often present with an 'acute-on-chronic' ischaemic picture, i.e., changes of acute ischaemia with some or more of the 6 Ps, but also with signs of chronic ischaemia.

Conclusion

A lower limb arterial duplex scan can be incredibly helpful in the assessment of vascular patients. Using the grey-scale function will enable you to visualise gross areas of pathology, and the colour Doppler and pulse wave Doppler functions can help you gain a more detailed understanding of arterial flow. The arterial duplex scan should always accompany a detailed history and examination of the patient and should naturally complement both your understanding of arterial anatomy and your appreciation of vascular pathology. This chapter focuses on 'normal' findings and indeed this should be your first area to get comfortable identifying on ultrasound. However, with increased practise and exposure to real clinical patients your experience will expand, and you will become more adept at identifying pathology using ultrasound.

CHAPTER 9
VENOUS ULTRASOUND

James M Forsyth

Learning Objectives

- Appreciate the relevant lower limb venous anatomy and common abbreviations for veins used in vascular surgery and interventional radiology settings.
- Have a basic understanding of the common pathologies affecting the lower limb venous system (specifically superficial venous reflux, varicose veins, venous leg ulcers, and deep vein thrombosis – DVT).
- Have a basic understanding of venous duplex scanning modalities including grey scale, colour Doppler and pulse wave Doppler.
- Be able to perform a basic lower limb venous duplex assessment.

In this chapter, I will briefly cover a vascular surgery point-of-care ultrasound assessment of the lower limb venous system. As with Chapter 8, this chapter represents an introduction into the world of venous duplex scanning. Venous disease and venous duplex scanning are specialist areas, and in this section the aim is to only explore the common and basic pathologies that are routinely encountered in everyday clinical settings. Again, in this chapter I have focussed on using wireless ultrasound technology, but the same principles apply when using standard ultrasound technology.

Anatomy

Superficial Veins

The two main superficial veins in the leg to consider are the great saphenous vein (GSV) and the small saphenous vein (SSV). *Note that sometimes the great saphenous vein is referred to as the long saphenous vein (LSV), and the small saphenous vein can be referred to as the short saphenous vein or lesser saphenous vein.* The GSV runs up the medial part of the leg towards the groin where it joins the common femoral vein (CFV) at the sapheno-femoral junction (SFJ). The small saphenous vein (SSV) runs up the back of the calf toward the popliteal fossa, where it joins the popliteal vein at the sapheno-popliteal junction (SPJ). See **Figure 9.1** for the relevant lower limb superficial venous anatomy.

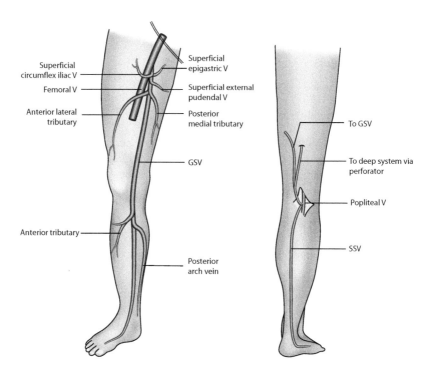

Figure 9.1 Basic lower limb superficial venous anatomy.

Deep Veins

The CFV is supplied by the femoral vein (FV) and the deep femoral (profunda) veins which are the main deep veins of the thigh. The FV is supplied by the popliteal vein, which is supplied by the distal calf veins (anterior tibial, posterior tibial and peroneal veins). These three distal calf veins are also considered to be deep veins although we will deliberately not focus on them in this introductory guide for the sake of simplicity. See **Figure 9.2** for the relevant lower limb deep venous anatomy.

***WARNING

In the past, the femoral vein was referred to as the *superficial femoral vein*. Many clinicians and ultrasonographers still use this nomenclature. However, this term should be avoided as it can lead clinicians to incorrectly assume it is not a deep vein, which can lead to confusion in the management of femoral vein thrombosis. It is easy to mistakenly think that a thrombus in the *superficial* femoral vein on an ultrasound report is not a deep vein thrombosis, and such a patient may not be treated as a DVT in such a context.

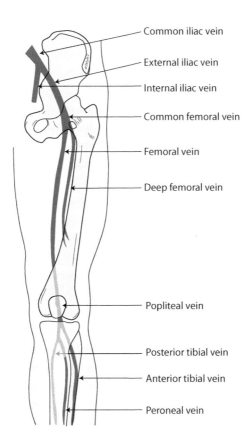

— Common iliac vein

— External iliac vein

— Internal iliac vein

— Common femoral vein

— Femoral vein

— Deep femoral vein

— Popliteal vein

— Posterior tibial vein

— Anterior tibial vein

— Peroneal vein

Figure 9.2 Basic lower limb deep venous anatomy.

Basic Lower Limb Venous Ultrasound Assessment

Preparation

■ Introduce yourself to the patient, explain the procedure and gain verbal consent.

■ Wash your hands and clean the ultrasound probe with an alcohol wipe.

■ Have a chaperone present throughout your assessment.

■ Ask the patient to take his/her trousers, shoes and socks off.

■ Position the patient in the standing upright position throughout your assessment. This is to aid venous filling and make your examination easier. Alternatively, the patient can lie on a bed that can be tilted feet-down/head-up.

Image Acquisition

GSV Assessment

■ Kneel or sit down in front of the patient who is standing facing you. Ask the patient to slightly retract their underwear upwards to allow you easier access into the groin crease. Also ask the patient to externally rotate his/her foot so the medial thigh/calf is more accessible.

■ In grey-scale function and with the ultrasound probe in transverse section, adjust your depth, gain and focus and manoeuvre the probe so you can identify the SFJ at the level of the groin crease. You should be able to see a 'Mickey Mouse' appearance of the CFA, CFV and GSV (see **Figure 9.3**). If you manoeuvre your probe in either longitudinal or transverse section, you will be able to identify the SFJ in greater detail (see **Figure 9.4**).

■ At this point, choose the pulse wave Doppler function. Drag the pointer so it lies over the SFJ, and visualise the SFJ in longitudinal section. Squeeze the patient's calf/lower thigh to force venous blood upwards through the junction. Assess to see if there is gross reflux (see **Figure 9.5**).

■ Continue to scan the GSV down toward the lower calf. In grey-scale function you can assess the size of the GSV, compressibility, tortuosity, etc. Note that a GSV diameter >5 mm has the best positive predictive value for pathological reflux (see **Figure 9.6**). You can use the pulse wave Doppler function in longitudinal section to further assess for incompetence (see **Figure 9.7**).

■ You can also use the Colour doppler function to examine for reflux. As you squeeze the leg you should see colour flow as the venous blood moves up towards the patient's heart. However, there should not be significant reversed colour flow coming back down the leg. This would indicate refluxing valves in the venous segment you are assessing.

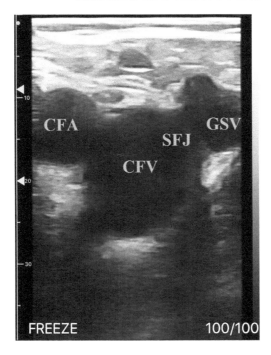

Figure 9.3 Ultrasound image showing confluence of GSV and CFV, with adjacent CFA. This gives a typical 'Mickey Mouse' appearance and represents the classic appearance of the sapheno-femoral junction (SFJ).

SSV Assessment

- Kneel or sit down in front of the patient who is now standing facing opposite you (i.e., their back is towards you).
- With the ultrasound probe in transverse or longitudinal section, adjust your depth, gain and focus and manoeuvre the probe so you can identify the SPJ in the popliteal fossa. You should be able to see the SSV diving deep to join the popliteal vein at the back of the knee (see **Figures 9.8** and **9.9**).
- At this point select the pulse wave Doppler function (or colour Doppler depending on your preference). At this point gently squeeze the patient's lower calf to force venous blood upwards through the junction. Assess to see if there is reflux, following exactly the same principles as with the SFJ/GSV assessment.
- Continue to scan the SSV down toward the ankle. In grey-scale function you can identify the size of the SSV and assess for compressibility, tortuosity, etc. Note that for pathological reflux of the

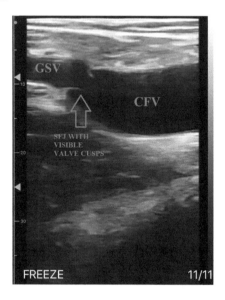

Figure 9.4 Focus on the SFJ in longitudinal section showing the actual valve cusps, where the GSV enters the CFV.

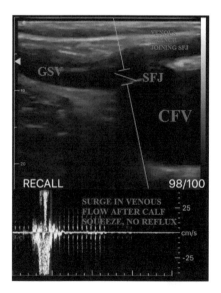

Figure 9.5 Longitudinal ultrasound image of normal healthy patient with no reflux demonstrated. As one squeezes the leg, there is a sudden rush of venous blood through the SFJ, which is represented by the sudden surge in flow. However, as the SFJ valve is functioning, there is no continued flow backwards and the flow suddenly ceases.

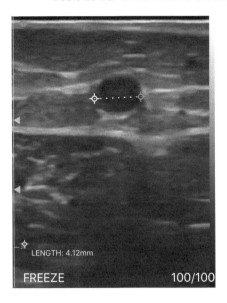

LENGTH: 4.12mm

FREEZE   100/100

Figure 9.6 Ultrasound image of normal healthy patient with GSV diameter of <5 mm (in transverse section).

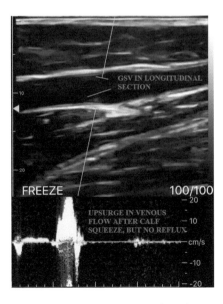

GSV IN LONGITUDINAL SECTION

10

20

FREEZE   100/100

UPSURGE IN VENOUS FLOW AFTER CALF SQUEEZE, BUT NO REFLUX

cm/s

Figure 9.7 Pulse wave Doppler being used to assess for reflux in the GSV (in longitudinal section). In this healthy patient no reflux was demonstrated.

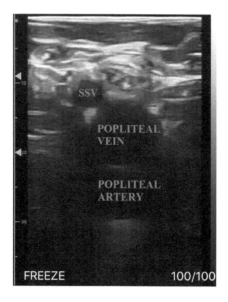

Figure 9.8 Transverse orientation showing the SSV diving down towards the popliteal vein which is lying directly above the popliteal artery.

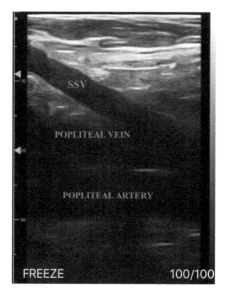

Figure 9.9 Longitudinal orientation showing the SSV diving down towards the popliteal vein (again with popliteal artery lying underneath the vein).

SSV, the best cut-off diameter is 3.5 mm (see **Figure 9.10**). Again, you can also use the pulse wave Doppler or colour Doppler to assess for SSV incompetence.

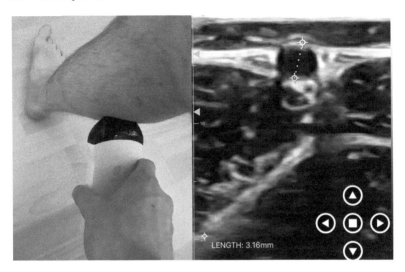

LENGTH: 3.16mm

Figure 9.10 Operator holding wireless probe in transverse section over upper posterior calf in order to visualise and measure width of SSV.

Deep Vein Assessment for Acute DVT

- I propose a simple grey-scale compression assessment of the proximal deep veins in three positions – at the groin, in the mid-thigh and behind the knee. For DVT assessment, use the ultrasound probe in *transverse section*. If you use transverse section, you can confidently visualise if the vein fully compresses or not, whereas using the ultrasound probe in longitudinal section makes it more difficult to visualise the complete compression process. For more complex DVT and calf vein scanning, please refer to specialist texts.

- Wherever possible the legs should be examined in a dependent position in order to distend the veins as much as possible and aid visualisation. Ideally, the legs should be tilted downward by at least 30° (reverse Trendelenburg position). Alternatively, the patient can be examined in the standing position.

- Use the wireless probe in transverse section and firstly assess the groin. Identify the 'Mickey Mouse' as described before, and compress the CFV. The walls of the CFV will easily and completely compress if there is no DVT (see **Figure 9.11** which shows CFV being compressed and CFA lying adjacent to it).

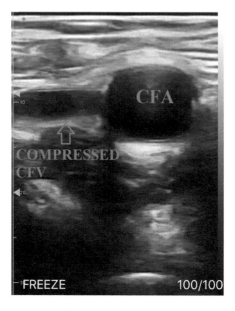

Figure 9.11 CFV that is easy to fully compress excludes DVT at this point. In this freeze frame, the CFV is almost fully compressed whilst the CFA remains patent.

- Repeat this step to reassess the CFV for a few centimetres upwards (towards the external iliac vein at the level of the inguinal ligament). Check for normal compressibility.
- Return to the 'Mickey Mouse' position, and then repeat the step again for a few centimetres downward to cover the origins of the femoral vein and the profunda femoral vein (see **Figures 9.12–9.14**). Check that they compress fully and easily.
- Now move your attention to the mid-thigh. Identify the SFA and the FV in transverse section and press downward with your ultrasound probe to compress the FV. A normal FV should easily compress, whilst the SFA should still be seen to be pulsating. Scan for a few centimetres above and below this point, again confirming normal compressibility of the FV.
- Finally, move your attention to the popliteal fossa. Again, use your wireless probe in transverse section to identify the popliteal vein in the mid-popliteal fossa. Confirm normal compressibility for a few centimetres above and below this point.
- You will need to calculate the patient's Wells score and also have the D-dimer result available. Of note, 'Likely' patients who have a positive D-dimer result but a negative proximal DVT ultrasound will require a repeat ultrasound scan of the proximal veins one week later.

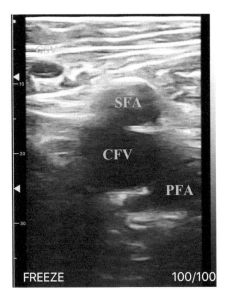

Figure 9.12 SFA, PFA, CFV and GSV all visible as the wireless probe moves downwards from the 'Mickey Mouse' position to identify origins of femoral and profunda femoral vein.

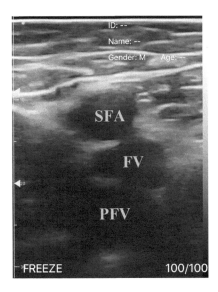

Figure 9.13 Normal femoral and profunda femoral vein as they split off from the CFV. At this point, the PFA has dived deep into the thigh and is not easily visible on the screen, but the SFA is easily apparent.

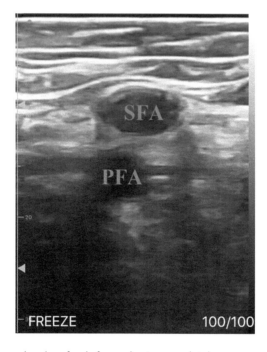

Figure 9.14 Femoral and profunda femoral veins completely compressed, now revealing SFA and PFA alone which have been forced closer together by the downward probe pressure. This confirms there is no thrombus in these normal sections of femoral and profunda femoral veins.

- At all times follow your clinical intuition, and remember that if you have any doubt or clinical concerns you can seek vascular surgery/interventional radiology for advice. For example, in the case of a patient with high clinical suspicion for DVT, a grossly swollen leg, but a negative proximal DVT ultrasound, the author would recommend discussing the case with vascular surgery/interventional radiology for a specialist opinion, possibly with specialist imaging to look for iliac or pelvic vein thrombosis or pelvic pathology that could be causing proximal venous compression.

Closing Steps

- Once you have completed your assessment, thank the patient and help remove the ultrasound gel from his/her skin.
- Wash your hands and cleanse the ultrasound probe with an alcohol wipe.
- Document your findings.
- Discuss your findings with the patient.
- Decide upon further investigations/treatments as necessary.

Common Pathology Affecting Venous System

The two most common clinical indications for assessing the lower limbs in a venous context are:

1. Varicose veins/venous leg ulceration
2. Deep vein thrombosis (DVT)

Superficial Venous Incompetence/Varicose Veins

If the superficial venous valves stop functioning it results in venous blood pooling under gravity around the ankles (causing venous hypertension), which can lead to the following signs and symptoms:

- Telangiectasia/spider veins
- Varicose veins (asymptomatic)
- Varicose veins (symptomatic, i.e., with discomfort/pain)
- Leg swelling/oedema
- Venous skin changes, i.e., eczema/pigmentation
- Venous ulceration
- Thrombophlebitis
- Bleeding varicose veins
- *Note*: GSV incompetence causes varicose veins around the inner thigh/calf with ulceration classically around the medial gaiter area/medial malleolus. SSV incompetence causes varicose veins around the posterior calf region with ulcers around the lateral malleolus.

Acute DVT

If there is acute thrombus within the deep veins of the lower limb, this can result in the following signs and symptoms:

- Calf warmth/tenderness/swelling/erythema
- Mild fever
- Pitting oedema

If the proximal deep veins are obstructed, this can present with a very swollen thigh as well as the calf (i.e., an ileofemoral DVT). *Phlegmasia alba dolens* is the swollen 'white' painful limb that is found in patients with ileofemoral DVT. These patients generally have a more limited occlusion of the iliac veins. *Phlegmasia cerulea dolens* is the swollen 'blue' painful limb that is seen in patients with a more significant ileofemoral DVT with more extensive thrombosis. In these patients, the venous hypertension is more pronounced with elevated compartment pressures leading to a greater degree of pain and discomfort. The blue cyanotic discolouration is caused by a stagnation of venous blood in the dermal and subdermal venous plexuses. At the most severe end of the spectrum is venous gangrene, which represents soft tissue necrosis in a limb with a large burden proximal DVT. This presentation usually represents a progression from *phlegmasia alba dolens* through *phlegmasia cerulea dolens*. The venous gangrene itself ultimately results from small vein and microvascular thrombosis. Venous gangrene in these contexts is often associated with malignancy and other serious conditions like heparin-induced thrombocytopenia, disseminated intravascular coagulation, acute liver dysfunction, and sepsis. Ileofemoral DVT should therefore be taken seriously and early consultation with vascular surgery is recommended.

Conclusion

Venous disease is a vast specialist area, and entire textbooks are devoted to it. However, this chapter hopes to cover the major areas that are encountered in day-to-day clinical practice. It must be emphasised that the clinical history and examination are the most important steps in the work-up of suspected venous disease. Likewise, an understanding of the relevant lower venous anatomy is of paramount importance. In simplistic terms, you should use the clinical history and examination findings to identify where you think the venous pathology is (e.g., GSV or SSV reflux) and use the ultrasound scanner to confirm or refute your diagnosis. In the context of a suspected DVT, the same principles apply. The clinical presentation and relevant biochemical results (i.e., D-dimer) should be sought first, and the ultrasound comes afterwards to confirm or refute your diagnosis. This chapter does not cover other more specialist areas of venous disease (e.g., deep venous reflux, deep venous obstruction, calf vein DVT scanning); however, if you can grasp the principles in this chapter, it will hopefully establish a foundation for further specialist training to advance upon.

PART III
ASSESSMENT

CHAPTER 10

SINGLE BEST ANSWER ASSESSMENT

1 How Does Ultrasound Work?

1.1. Medical ultrasound operates over which frequency range?
   A. 2–20 MHz
   B. 0–10 Hz
   C. 20–100 kHz
   D. 10–20,000 Hz
   E. 20–100 MHz

1.2. Which tissue has the lowest impedance to ultrasound?
   A. Bone
   B. Lung
   C. Liver
   D. Tendon
   E. Blood

1.3. What does the Doppler effect describe for a moving sound source relative to a stationary observer?
   A. An increase in detected volume when moving towards the observer
   B. A decrease in detected volume when moving away from the observer
   C. An increase in detected frequency when moving towards the observer
   D. An increase in detected frequency when moving away from the observer
   E. A decrease in the detected frequency when moving towards the observer

1.4. Which type of ultrasound transducer would be best suited to imaging of the heart (echocardiography)?
   A. 3.5–5 MHz convex probe
   B. 7.5–10 MHz linear probe
   C. 3–5 MHz phased array probe
   D. 10–14 MHz linear probe
   E. 3.5–5 MHz micro-convex probe

1.5. A foundation doctor has been asked to place a peripheral venous cannula in a patient in whom access has been difficult in the past. He decides to use ultrasound to identify a suitable peripheral vein and selects a linear probe with a frequency range of 5–14 MHz. He locates what he thinks is a suitable cephalic vein in the right forearm with a frequency setting on his probe of 7.5 MHz but the image is blurred and indistinct. What should he do to improve the resolution of the image?

A. Select a lower-frequency setting
B. Select a higher-frequency setting
C. Turn up the gain
D. Adjust the focus
E. Adjust the depth

1.6. What are the physical effects of ultrasound on tissues and what corresponding rating helps maintain these effects within safe limits?

A. Tissue heating, mechanical index (MI)
B. Cavitation, thermal index (TI)
C. Tissue heating, thermal index (TI)
D. Tissue radiation damage, millisievert (mSv)
E. Genotoxicity due to electromagnetic field, magnetic flux density (Nm/A)

2 POCUS

2.1. A 24-year-old male pedestrian has been involved in an RTA where he received high impact trauma to his right upper abdomen and chest. Which POCUS protocol would be most appropriate in this case?

A. FAST
B. FEEL
C. BLUE
D. eFAST
E. RUSH

2.2. You are a member of the cardiac arrest team and have been called to the medical admissions unit where the medical team is attending a 65-year-old male who is peri-arrest. Admitted 4 hours previously with worsening breathlessness and hypotension, this patient was treated with fluid resuscitation but had failed to improve. His past medical history is unremarkable. His chest radiograph on admission showed cardiomegaly and bilateral pleural effusions. How might POCUS be best employed in this scenario?

A. Thoracic ultrasound to tap the pleural effusions
B. Ultrasound for exploration of peripheral venous access
C. FEEL protocol to assess for reversible causes of cardiac arrest
D. Ultrasound guided placement of central line
E. Abdominal ultrasound examination to explore possible source of sepsis

2.3. You are working on the high dependency unit and are responsible for the care of a 75-year-old female admitted with a severe community acquired pneumonia and sepsis. She has a blood pressure of 80/40 mmHg, pulse 140/min, temperature 38°C, and a urine output of less than 15 mL/hour despite aggressive fluid resuscitation. She requires high flow nasal oxygen and inotropic support. How do you assess fluid status?

A. Examine skin turgor and if JVP is not raised then give a further fluid challenge
B. Increase inotropic support
C. Carry out a thoracic ultrasound to exclude empyema
D. Use bedside ultrasound to image the IVC for respiratory collapse
E. Assess LV function using micro-bubble contrast echocardiography

2.4. You are the doctor for a football club. One of the players is injured and complains of sudden onset pain just above his right heel (posteriorly). He is having difficulty bearing his weight and is clearly in pain. He has been stretchered off and you are asked to assess his injury and advise on further management. Which course of action would be best?

A. Rub down the ankle with a warm sponge and recommend return to the field of play.
B. Examine the ankle for swelling and pain on plantar extension; if findings are positive then place an elasticated bandage and recommend rest.
C. Apply an ice pack and arrange an MRI examination for the following day.
D. Carry out an ultrasound assessment of the Achilles tendon, looking for a discontinuity in the tendon and surrounding oedema; if positive, arrange for urgent splinting and orthopaedic review.
E. Carry out a Doppler ultrasound of the calf to look for a deep vein thrombosis.

Single Best Answer Assessment

3 Neck Ultrasound

3.1. Which of these salivary glands is positioned just anterior to the ear?
  A. Parotid gland
  B. Submandibular gland
  C. Sublingual gland
  D. Thyroid gland
  E. Parathyroid gland(s)

3.2. How many nodal levels are there in the neck?
  A. 3
  B. 4
  C.. 5
  D. 6
  E. 7

3.3. Which type of probe is most suitable for ultrasound of the neck?
  A. Curvilinear probe, low frequency
  B. Curvilinear probe, high frequency
  C. Linear probe, low frequency
  D. Linear probe, high frequency
  E. Microconvex probe, low frequency

3.4. Which of these imaging features is NOT concerning for malignancy in a neck lymph node?
  A. Increased vascularity
  B. Ovoid shape
  C. Heterogenous echotexture
  D. Large size
  E. Clumping of several nodes together

4 Thoracic Ultrasound

4.1. B-lines on an ultrasound scan of the lung are:
  A. Horizontal lines representing pleural reverberation artefact
  B. Vertical lines radiating from the pleura representing interstitial oedema
  C. Bright lines which 'slide' with respiration
  D. Bright lines superficial to the intercostal space
  E. Caused by pleural effusion

4.2. You are a GP on a remote Scottish island and have been asked to see a young male smoker who is of tall, thin body habitus. He presents with sudden onset left-sided chest pain and difficulty in taking a deep breath. You do not have access to x-ray facilities which would require a 5-hour ferry or half-hour helicopter journey to the closest medical facility. You have a hand-held ultrasound scanner and are keen to confidently discriminate musculoskeletal chest pain from a significant left-sided pneumothorax. When carrying out a thoracic ultrasound examination, what would you specifically look for?

A. Multiple B-lines
B. Multiple A-lines
C. Absence of lung sliding and the 'barcode sign' in M-mode
D. Lung consolidation
E. Absent diaphragmatic movement

4.3. You have been referred a 70-year-old retired joiner with weight loss and worsening breathlessness. His past medical history includes a previous myocardial infarction within the last year. His chest x-ray shows right lower zone opacification in keeping with a large pleural effusion. What would be the next best diagnostic step?

A. Prescribe diuretics and repeat the chest radiograph in 2 weeks
B. Arrange for a computed tomography (CT) scan
C. Insert an intercostal drain and send fluid for biochemical analysis
D. Carry out thoracocentesis and send samples of fluid to Cytology
E. Carry out a detailed pleural ultrasound and aspirate fluid under ultrasound guidance for further testing.

5 Cardiac Ultrasound

5.1. Echocardiography and Pulmonary Embolus
Choose the *most* correct answer.

A. TOE will readily image the main, right and left pulmonary artery in ventilated patients suspected to have suffered a PE.
B. TTE features of pulmonary embolus include a dilated right heart, RV hypokinesia, pulmonary hypertension, RV thrombus and ventricular interdependence.
C. If performing echocardiography among haemodynamically unstable patients with suspected PE, unequivocal signs of RV pressure overload and dysfunction justifies reperfusion therapy.
D. Akinesia of the mid-ventricular RV with hyper-contractility of the RV apex is McDonalds sign.
E. RV dilation is found in over 50% of patients with PE.

5.2. Echocardiography in Cardiac Tamponade
   A. Diagnosis depends on the collapse of the right atrium and ventricle in diastole.
   B. Diagnosis depends on the collapse of the right ventricle and respiratory variation of mitral/tricuspid Doppler inflows.
   C. Diagnosis depends on clinical findings of hypotension, tachycardia, elevated JVP and at least a moderate pericardial effusion.
   D. The diagnosis is clinical and the patient may be in cardiac tamponade without echocardiographic features.
   E. Can occur in aortic dissection necessitating emergency percutaneous drainage.

6 Abdomino-Pelvic Ultrasound

6.1. An 84-year-old male is admitted with a history of weight loss and lethargy. He was recently discharged following surgery for prostate cancer. Analysis of blood results showed him to have an acute kidney injury. You suspect an obstructive nephropathy and therefore carry out a point-of-care ultrasound of the kidneys. Which diagnostic features are you looking for?
   A. An anechoic area in the renal pelvis and calyceal dilatation
   B. Horseshoe-shaped kidney
   C. Reduced kidney size
   D. Contraction of renal calyces
   E. Parenchymal thickening

6.2. With regard to the ultrasound examination of the liver, how many liver segments are there?
   A. 2
   B. 4
   C. 6
   D. 8
   E. 10

6.3. What could you do to improve your view of the liver?
   A. Ask the patient to roll onto his side
   B. Change to a linear probe
   C. Ask the patient to breathe in
   D. Increase your frequency
   E. Ask the patient to lie prone

6.4. How should a patient prepare for their ultrasound if the clinical question is gallstones?
A. Fill their bladder
B. Fast for 12 hours
C. Fast for 6 hours
D. Eat something immediately prior to the examination
E. Fast for 4 hours

7 Musculoskeletal Ultrasound

7.1. Which of these is *NOT* a muscle of the rotator cuff?
A. Supraspinatus
B. Infraspinatus
C. Subscapularis
D. Teres major
E. Teres minor

7.2. What type of probe is most suitable for musculoskeletal ultrasound?
A. Curvilinear probe, low frequency
B. Curvilinear probe, high frequency
C. Linear probe, low frequency
D. Linear probe, high frequency
E. Phased array probe, intermediate frequency

8 Vascular Ultrasound

8.1. A 79-year-old non-smoking gentleman presents with a 4-hour history of sudden onset left foot pain and discolouration. He is known to have atrial fibrillation, and is not currently anticoagulated because of a high falls risk. On examination he has a strong femoral pulse in the left groin but no pulses distally. All his pulses are palpable on the right side. His left foot is cool and pale, and he has absent sensation in his toes, with reduced sensation in the forefoot. He can also barely move his toes. His left calf is soft and non-tender. Using your ultrasound probe you visualise normal CFA, SFA and PFA origins with normal colour Doppler flow. As you advance down the SFA in the longitudinal section it appears grossly normal, when all of a sudden in the lower-thigh section, the colour Doppler flow signal ceases and the artery stops pulsating. Which of the following statements is correct?

A. This gentleman has acute-on-chronic arterial disease. His foot is not threatened and he can be managed conservatively.

B. The most likely cause of this patient's symptoms is acute thrombotic occlusion of his below knee popliteal artery.

C. In the context of this clinical picture the reduced sensation and reduced power in his foot are not concerning clinical signs.

D. This gentleman has acute embolic ischaemia secondary to atrial fibrillation. His foot is threatened but viable and he requires immediate revascularisation.

E. This gentleman has acute embolic ischaemia secondary to atrial fibrillation. His foot is non-viable and he requires either a major amputation or palliation.

8.2. A 64-year-old gentleman is brought into the emergency department by the paramedics. Apart from well-controlled hypertension this gentleman is otherwise fit and well. He collapsed at home and is now complaining of severe back pain. On examination you think you can feel a pulsatile expansile abdominal mass; however, as the patient is slightly overweight you are not completely confident that this is an AAA. The patient is profoundly shocked with a systolic blood pressure of 68 mmHg and a heart rate of 130. He looks peri-arrest and has a Glasgow Coma Score (GCS) of 13/15. You use your low/intermediate-frequency wireless ultrasound probe to scan the patient's abdomen, and identify an 8.6 cm AAA. You are in a district hospital with no vascular surgery support on-site, and the nearest tertiary vascular unit is about a 10-minute drive away (via blue-light ambulance). Which of the following statements is correct?

A. This clinical presentation suggests a symptomatic AAA.

B. This clinical presentation suggests a ruptured AAA. The patient should be sent for an urgent CT scan to confirm your diagnosis, and discussed with the on-site general surgical team.

C. This clinical presentation suggests a ruptured AAA. The patient should be discussed with the nearest on-call vascular surgery team with a view to urgent transfer to them. During the ambulance transfer he can be transfused 0-negative blood to maintain his conscious level, aiming for a systolic blood pressure of 70–80 mmHg.

D. This clinical presentation suggests acute pancreatitis or a perforated abdominal viscus. The patient requires an urgent upright chest x-ray and amylase testing along with an urgent general surgical review.

E. This patient should be transfused multiple blood products and aggressively fluid resuscitated immediately (to achieve a normal blood pressure of 120/80 mmHg).

8.3. An 80-year-old male patient comes to see you (his community physician) in your rural community practice. The patient is complaining of severe pain in his right foot and toes that is present all the time. He is struggling to sleep at night and is now forced to sleep sitting up in a chair. He has also developed a small ulcer on the great toe. These new symptoms started about 3 weeks ago. He also says that when he walks about 20 m he gets severe calf pain that forces him to stop. He has been getting this calf pain for years but it has been gradually worsening. On examination you can only feel a faint femoral pulse, but nothing distally. Using your wireless ultrasound probe you identify a heavily diseased common femoral artery with significantly reduced colour flow. The patient's superficial femoral artery also appears to have a number of areas of stenotic disease. Which of the following statements is correct?

A. This clinical picture is most likely explained by the diagnosis of sciatica.

B. This clinical picture suggests a diagnosis of acute limb ischaemia secondary to an embolic event.

C. This clinical picture suggests chronic limb-threatening ischaemia. The patient should be advised to stop smoking and discharged with no further follow-up.

D. This patient should be referred non-urgently to an orthopaedic surgeon with a specialist interest in foot and ankle disease for suspected gout.

E. This patient has chronic limb-threatening ischaemia with tissue loss. He needs to stop smoking, be commenced upon an antiplatelet agent and cholesterol-lowering therapy and referred urgently to a vascular surgeon.

8.4. You are a foundation doctor currently working in community medicine. You are doing a home visit for a 60-year-old female patient who suffers from chronic back problems and obesity. She has mobility issues and has therefore been unable to come to the clinic for a while. She is also a heavy smoker. You have been called out to see her urgently because of a painful leg ulcer. The ulcer is placed around her lower posterior calf on the right leg. The skin surrounding the ulcer is slightly erythematous and warm to touch, and it is slightly smelly. The patient also has palpable varicosities around the back of her knee, and she has a chronic brownish pigmentation around the lower leg. Wireless ultrasound assessment of the lower leg reveals a normal-sized GSV, with no obvious reflux. However, the SSV is demonstrating obvious reflux. The patient is systemically well with normal clinical observation parameters. Which of the following statements is correct?

A. This clinical presentation suggests SSV distribution venous reflux causing a venous leg ulcer that can currently be managed with oral antibiotics. Before compression therapy can be applied her arterial system should be assessed also. She should be referred to a vascular surgeon for further assessment.

B. This clinical presentation suggests acute limb ischaemia secondary to acute thrombotic occlusion of the SFA.

C. This clinical presentation suggests GSV distribution venous reflux causing a venous leg ulcer that requires urgent admission to hospital for intravenous antibiotics.

D. This clinical presentation suggests SSV distribution venous reflux causing a venous leg ulcer that should be treated with compression therapy and can be managed in the community.

E. This clinical presentation primarily suggests chronic limb threatening ischaemia with tissue loss.

Answers

1 How Does Ultrasound Work?

1.1. A

1.2. B

1.3. C

1.4. C

1.5. B

1.6. C

2 POCUS

2.1. D

2.2. C

2.3. D

2.4. D

3 Neck Ultrasound

3.1. A

3.2. E

3.3. D

3.4. B

4 Thoracic Ultrasound

4.1. B

4.2. C

4.3. E

5 Cardiac Ultrasound

5.1. C

- Echocardiography should be used routinely to assess haemodynamically unstable patients. It will exclude other cardiac causes such as LV dysfunction or tamponade and can assess fluid status. CTPA is not possible in unstable patients, and so RV pressure load without other causes of hypotension justifies emergency treatment in patients suspected to have had massive PE.
- TOE does not readily image the left pulmonary artery, but is useful in ventilated patients.
- Ventricular interdependence is a sign of constrictive physiology.
- D describes McConnell's sign.
- 143RV dilation is found in over 25% patients with PE. Therefore it should not be used routinely in the assessment of PE.

5.2. D

Cardiac tamponade is a clinical diagnosis and a medical/surgical emergency. In most modern-day clinical settings, there is time to perform emergency echocardiography and this should be done whenever possible. Answers (A) and (B) describe echocardiographic features of cardiac tamponade but without the clinical context. Rapid accumulation of a small amount of pericardial fluid can cause tamponade. Slow accumulation of a massive amount of fluid may not cause tamponade. A loculated effusion can cause tamponade without the classical echocardiographic features. Cardiac tamponade in the setting of aortic dissection is a surgical emergency and should be treated with emergency thoracotomy.

6 Abdomino-Pelvic Ultrasound

6.1. A

6.2. D

6.3. C

6.4. E

7 Musculoskeletal Ultrasound

7.1. D

7.2. D

8 Vascular Ultrasound

8.1. D

This patient has acute embolic occlusion of his left SFA secondary to atrial fibrillation. The reduced power and sensation in his foot means his leg is threatened. Absent power and sensation, with fixed mottling of the skin and a tender rigid calf muscle would suggest irreversible ischaemia, which he does not yet have.

8.2. C

A symptomatic AAA is when the aneurysm is not ruptured but is causing the patient pain (i.e., a tender aneurysm, back pain, abdominal pain. etc., in the absence of other obvious causes). Symptomatic AAAs are deemed to be at a high risk of rupture, therefore are still considered to be a vascular surgery emergency. However, this case is clearly a ruptured AAA. The AAA has clearly burst and is leading to haemorrhagic shock. In the author's opinion in this context the patient should not go to the CT scanner. His best chances of survival are instead to be sent immediately to the nearest vascular surgery unit. When (if) he reaches the vascular team they can decide if he requires a CT scan. Involving the general surgical team in this patient's care is unnecessary and would only lead to further time delays. Also transfusing gallons of blood/crystalloids will likely lead to a worse outcome. You should be aiming to achieve 'permissive hypotension'. Fluid resuscitation should be sufficient to maintain consciousness, and in the shocked AAA patient you should aim for systolic pressures of 70–80 mmHg. Aggressive volume resuscitation prior to aortic control is a predictor of increased post-operative mortality. If you have blood available it should accompany the patient during transfer and can be given to maintain consciousness.

8.3. E

This patient has chronic limb-threatening disease with tissue loss. This will almost certainly have been caused by atherosclerosis that is likely secondary to a chronic heavy smoking history. This is a vascular surgery emergency and the patient requires urgent referral to a vascular surgeon for consideration of revascularisation in order to prevent limb loss. The ultrasound result clearly indicates this patient has vascular disease, and the disease is multi-level. Indeed all such patients should be on best medical therapy and advised to stop smoking.

8.4. A

This woman's symptoms primarily suggest SSV distribution venous reflux which explains why the varicosities are in the posterior calf and the ulcer is around the lateral malleolus. Anatomically this reflects the course of the SSV. As she has an ulcer this represents severe venous disease and she should therefore be referred to a vascular surgeon for ongoing investigation and management. It would be unwise to place her in compression therapy without confirming she has normal foot pulses and/or a normal ankle-brachial pressure index (ABPI). The leg ulcer seems like it is infected but as she is systemically well a trial of oral antibiotics would be a sensible first approach.

INDEX

Index

Index

T - #0661 - 071024 - C170 - 216/138/8 - PB - 9780367349585 - Gloss Lamination